POSITIVE PRACTICE

POSITIVE PRACTICE
A Step-by-Step Guide to Family Therapy

Alan Carr

Department of Psychology
University College Dublin
and
The Clanwilliam Institute, Dublin

h○
ap

harwood academic publishers

Austria • Australia • Belgium • France • Germany • India • Japan • Malaysia
Netherlands • Russia • Singapore • Switzerland • Thailand • United Kingdom • USA

Harwood Academic Publishers
Poststrasse 22
7000 Chur, Switzerland

British Library Cataloguing in Publication Data

Carr, Alan
  Positive practice:Step-by-step Guide to
  Family Therapy
  I. Title
  616.89156

  ISBN 3-7186-5678-7 (Hardcover)
  ISBN 3-7186-5680-9 (Softcover)

CONTENTS

FOREWORD

As a professor in a graduate programme in marriage and family therapy, I have long thought it critical to train student therapists using step-by-step methods, clearly articulating the specifics necessary in doing family therapy. Almost every other health-care discipline trains their practitioners that way. Psychotherapy in general, and family therapy in particular, seems reluctant to propose a *method* of fundamental practice to students and then teach them how to do it. Instead we insist that all models of therapy be taught at the beginning, and assume the student will eventually develop his or her own "style" of therapy. Although I think students do eventually learn to do therapy using this approach, I think it is often an awkward frustrating process which could be improved upon greatly using more systematic techniques.

With that rather strong opinion about family therapy training, imagine my delight when I read *Positive Practice*. Dr Carr has developed precisely the type of book which offers such a step-by-step approach for new family therapy practitioners. It is really more of a treatment manual than the typical professional therapy book. *Positive Practice* gives specific, detailed instructions on how to conduct family therapy, from initial contact, through assessment, through treatment planning, through intervention, through final evaluation. This book offers a point-by-point, session-by-session formulation for treatment which students will find extremely helpful.

The book is rich with clinical examples which will also help the beginning therapist more fully integrate the material. However, these are not "case-studies" per se, but instead short examples woven into the manual to help exemplify the point being made. I personally find this method the most useful. Also included are many clinical resources, such as sample letters, homework assignments, and metaphors which will also be of immediate use.

Because *Positive Practice* is practical and systematic in its presentation, this does not mean that it is atheoretical. On the contrary, Dr Carr from the beginning offers his underlying theory of clinical practice. In fact, the title of the book also is the theory of practice, which is a model integrating Milan systems, psychodynamic and social learning theories. However, unlike the latter two theories, Positive Practice is informed to a great extent from social-constructionism. The *family's* view of the problem, as well as their view of the solution, is critical in this model. At the same time, while the underlying theory is certainly clear, it is not imposing. Those who find the pragmatics of clinical practice more useful than theoretical discussions will most appreciate this book.

Positive Practice, by the way, should not be viewed simply for beginning therapists. I have been practicing for......well, a few years myself, and found not only many new ideas but also a reminder of how to conceptualize family consultation using the "big picture". I think experienced therapists, who would honestly have to admit that they do therapy more by the "seat of their pants", will also find this book quite useful, both as a basic review and as offering a new framework for organizing their cases. The troubleshooting sections will prove exceptionally helpful to newer and more seasoned therapists alike.

Positive Practice is quite accessible, being both well-written and well-organized. I would recommend a beginning family therapist use this as a formal treatment manual; that is, use it almost verbatim, session-by-session. It will prove to be both practical and comforting. It is practical, because it will guide the student through most of the combinations and permutations of therapist–client interaction and still guide the course of effective treatment. It is comforting, because it will give the beginning family therapist the blueprint and the materials to manage the course of therapy.

I think you will truly enjoy this important and highly original work. Dr Carr should be congratulated on both the effort and the result.

I am hopeful that this book may usher in an era of more treatment manual approaches to clinical training. The students will certainly appreciate it, and ultimately their clients will as well.

Terry S. Trepper, PhD
Director of Family Studies Centre and Professor of Psychology
Purdue University Calumet
Editor of the *Journal of Family Psychotherapy* and
Senior Editor of the *Haworth Series on Marriage and the Family*.

PREFACE

This book is for newcomers to the field of family therapy and systemic consultation. It describes an approach to consultation and therapy which may be used when children or adolescents are referred with social or psychological problems. The approach may be used in both public and private agencies by professionals from a variety of disciplines including psychology, psychiatry, social work, nursing, occupational therapy, paediatrics and general medical practice. This book is written as a treatment manual and as a training resource for professionals wishing to adopt this style of practice, and for trainers. For the sake of clarity, many diagrammatic conceptual frameworks and skills checklists have been included. Practical exercises are given at the end of each chapter. In most instances, the exercises require a small group of between two and eight professionals. For this reason, you may find it useful to work through the book reading a chapter at a time and reserving two hours per week to meet with a small group of colleagues or trainees to discuss the material and complete the exercises.

The approach to practice described here evolved in a particular context. The bulk of the model was explicitly formulated over a seven year period in the 1980s and early 1990s while working in a UK National Health Service Child and Family Clinic (Carr, McDonnell and Owen, 1994). During this period there was a national emphasis on cooperation between health service professionals and their colleagues in social services and education. There was also an emphasis on liaison between district hospital departments offering services to children such as child psychology, child psychiatry and paediatrics. In addition, many hospitals within the NHS became privately run trusts. These factors created a climate which favoured the development of models of assessment and intervention that were time limited, that took account of the wider professional network of which the child and therapist were part, which clearly addressed the overlap between the roles of therapist and agent of social control and which could be evaluated or audited in a relatively objective way.

The approach described in this book is called Positive Practice. It looks to the tradition of Milan systemic family therapy for its central clinical framework (Tomm, 1984a; b). Aspects of psychodynamic therapy (e.g. Malan, 1979) and social learning theory (e.g. Falloon, 1991) are integrated into this core approach to practice. The model, as a whole, is informed by empirical research on child development, social psychology, psychotherapy and the provision of mental health services (Carr, 1994a). This approach therefore, is part of the current integrationist movement within the field of family therapy (Breunlin, 1994). A central feature of Positive Practice is that the clinician explores ways of integrating new empirical findings, theoretical insights and practical procedures into a coherent, unified approach to consultation.

Many of us who work in the field of consultation and therapy at some time during our professional development hold the view that there is a *true formulation* of the client's problems and a related correct set of solutions. In Positive Practice this philosophical position, *naive realism*, is rejected. Rather, here it is assumed that the formulation which emerges from talking with children and parents about the presenting problem is no more than a construction. Since it is possible to construct multiple formulations to explain any problem, it is important to have a criterion by which to judge the merit of any particular one. In Positive Practice the *usefulness* of the formulation in suggesting a variety of feasible solutions which are acceptable to the family and the larger network of which it is part is the sole criterion for judging the merit of one formulation over another. Because of its emphasis on the socially constructed nature of problem-formulations and the choice of usefulness as a criterion for selecting between different formulations of the same problem, Positive Practice may be viewed as falling within the post-modernist traditions of social-constructionism and neopragmatism (Polkinghorne, 1992).

ACKNOWLEDGEMENTS

I am grateful to the many colleagues, friends and relatives who have helped me develop the ideas presented in this book. In particular I would like to thank the group who introduced me to family therapy at the Mater Hospital in Dublin in the late 1970s: Imelda McCarthy, Nollaig Byrne, Koos Mandos, Jim Sheehan and Paul McQuaid.

I am also grateful to Chris Cooper, Peter Simms and Carol Elisabeth Burra in Kingston, Ontario with whom I worked while living in Canada.

In the UK my gratitude goes to Steve Hunt and to the group with whom I practiced at Thurlow House and the Queen Elizabeth Hospital in King's Lynn during the 1980s and early 1990s: Dermot McDonnell, Chris Wood, George Gawlinski, Shiela Docking, Sue Grant, Nick Irving, Shahin Afnan, Jonathan Dossetor, Dennis Barter, Denise Sherwood and Mike Cliffe.

Thanks are due to John Carpenter, Bebe Speed and Bryan Lask at the editorial office of the *Journal of Family Therapy;* to Peter Stratton, editor of *Human Systems: The Journal of Systemic Consultation and Management;* to Max Cornwall who was editor at *The Australian Journal of Family Therapy* and to Terry Trepper, editor of *Journal of Family Psychotherapy* for challenging me to articulate my ideas more clearly.

Since returning to Ireland, my colleagues at UCD, particularly Thérèse Brady and Ciarán Benson, have been very supportive of my efforts to write this book. I am grateful to them for their encouragement and to Eunice McCarthy for her goodwill at a critical time in the development of these ideas.

For the gracious invitation to join their practice, a special word of thanks is due to my colleagues at the Clanwilliam Institute in Dublin: Ed McHale, Phil Kearney, Cory deJong, Declan Roche and Angela Walsh.

Much of what I know about family life I have learned from my own family, and to them I owe a particular debt of gratitude.

Go raibh míle maith agaibh go léir.

Alan Carr, May 1994

xi

"New worlds for old"

James Joyce (1922, *Ulysses*, p. 462)

"One beginning and one ending for a book was a thing I did not agree with. A good book may have three openings entirely dissimilar and inter-related only in the prescience of the author, or for that matter one hundred times as many endings...One book, one opening, was a principle with which I did not find it possible to concur."

Flann O'Brien (1939, *At Swim-two-birds*, pp. 9, 13)

1

Positive Practice as a Developmental and Recursive Process

Positive Practice may be viewed as both a developmental and a recursive process. It is a developmental process insofar as it consists of a series of distinct stages. At each stage key tasks must be completed before progression to the next stage. Failure to complete the tasks of a given stage before progressing to the next stage may jeopardise the consultation process. It is a recursive process insofar as it is possible to move from the final stage of one episode of consultation to the first stage of the next. The process is diagrammed in Figure 1.1. What follows is a description of the stages of consultation and the tasks entailed by each.

Stage 1. Planning Engagement

There are two main things that the therapist has to plan before the first session: (1) who to invite to this meeting and (2) what to talk to them about.

Stage 1.1. Planning who to invite

To make a plan about who to invite to the first session, the therapist must find out from the referral letter or through telephone contact who is involved with the problem and tentatively establish what roles they play with respect to it. With some cases this will be straightforward. But in others, it will be complex. In one instance, I was referred a family where over fifteen professionals were involved along with four foster parents. Positive Practice provides a system for mapping out the roles that each member of the problem system play. This is described in Chapter 2. Once each person's role has been established, decisions about who to invite to the intake session may be made. One particularly important role in the problem system is that of the customer. Customers are those members of the system most eager to see the problem resolved. Customers are always invited to the first session. The decision about who else to invite will depend upon the roles they are suspected to play in the problem system and their availability.

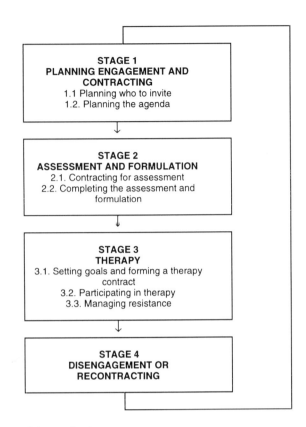

Figure 1.1.   Stages of the consultation process

Stage 1.2. Planning an agenda

In Positive Practice the therapist explicitly forms a preliminary formulation on the basis of the information in the referral letter or the referral telephone contact. This preliminary formulation or hypothesis is constructed according to a specific model. This three column formulation model, which is elaborated in Chapter 3, takes account of the current pattern of interaction around the presenting problem, the beliefs and other cognitive factors that constrain system members from breaking out of this problem-maintaining cycle of interaction, and historical events or other factors which underpin these constraining beliefs. The preliminary formulation or hypothesis provides the therapist with a number of avenues of questioning to pursue in the first interview when inquiring about the presenting problem, its evolution, maintenance and exceptional circumstances where the problem does not occur. The preliminary formulation also suggests areas where detailed inquiry is worthwhile when taking developmental and family histories and constructing a genogram.

Stage 2. Assessment and Formulation

Establishing a contract for assessment, working through the assessment agenda, developing a formulation on which to base treatment and trouble-shooting difficulties associated with non-attendance are the more important features of the assessment and formulation stage.

Stage 2.1. Establishing an assessment contract

At the outset of the assessment session the first task is to explain what assessment involves and to offer each member of the network a chance to accept or reject the opportunity to complete the assessment. For most parents, this will involve outlining the way in which the interviews will be conducted. The concept of a family interview with adjunctive individual interviews is unusual for many parents. Most parents need to be told about the time commitment required. An assessment may require between one and three sessions. It is important to highlight the voluntary nature of the assessment. It is also important to clarify the limits of confidentiality. Normally, the contents of sessions are confidential unless there is evidence that a family member is a serious threat to themselves or to others.

With children and teenagers, misconceptions need to be dispelled. For example, some children think that they will be admitted to hospital and others believe that they will be put in a detention centre. In some instances children may not wish to attend but their parents may be insistent. In others, parent's may not wish to attend but a referring physician or social worker may forcefully recommend attendance. In such situations, the therapist may facilitate the negotiation of some compromise between parties. For example, an agreement may be reached that a child will attend but not participate in the interview until the last fifteen minutes. If a cotherapy team is conducting the interview or a team and screen are in use, the roles of team members and the way in which the screen works needs to be explained. If sessions are to be videotaped, legally responsible guardians of children must sign the consent forms which stipulate the limits of use of these tapes. The contracting for assessment is complete when family members have been adequately informed about the process and have agreed to complete the assessment. Chapter 4 contains a detailed guide to the development of an assessment contract and also highlights ways of dealing with contracting problems.

Stage 2.2. Completing assessment and formulation

An assessment typically involves between one and three family interviews. These focus on working through the planned agenda developed in Stage 1.2 so that the therapist and the family may construct a three column formulation of the problem. The assessment is complete when the presenting problem and related difficulties are clarified, the cycles of social interaction within which these problems are embedded have been described, the factors that prevent involved members of the problem-system from breaking out of these cycles of interaction have been agreed upon, and exceptional circumstances where the problem does not occur have been identified. Exploring the child and family histories and constructing a genogram are typically employed as ways of bringing forth information useful for constructing the formulation. A detailed account of assessment procedures is presented in Chapters 5 and 6. The process of assessment also serves as a way for the family and therapist to form a working relationship, a relationship that will be vital for the success of therapy if the family opt for this.

Difficulties in engaging family members in the assessment process sometime occur and many of these are discussed in Chapter 2. Positive Practice offers ways for trouble shooting these difficulties. In some instances, the preliminary mapping of the problem-system may be at fault and, for example, the customer may have been misidentified. In other cases customers may require coaching on how to engage other family members in therapy.

Stage 3. Therapy

Once a formulation has been constructed the family may be invited to agree a contract for therapy, or it may be clear that therapy is unnecessary. In some cases, the process of assessment and formulation leads to problem resolution. Two patterns of assessment-based problem resolution are common. In the first, the problem is reframed so that the family no longer see it as a problem. For example, the problem is redefined as a normal reaction, a developmental phase or an unfortunate but transient incident. In the second, the process of assessment releases family members' natural problem-solving skills and they resolve the problem themselves. For example, many parents, once they discuss their anxiety about handling their child in a productive way during a family assessment interview, feel released to do so.

In other cases assessment leads on to contracting for an episode of therapy. Therapy rarely runs a smooth and predictable course, and the management of the difficulties and impasses that develop in the midphase of therapy is an important aspect of Positive Practice.

Stage 3.1. Setting goals and forming a therapy contract

The contracting process involves presenting a clear formulation of the problem, establishing clearly defined and realistic goals and outlining a plan to work towards those goals. Ways of managing this process are discussed in Chapter 7. Of all of these tasks, goal-setting is the most vital. Clear, realistic, visualised goals that are fully accepted by all family members are crucial for effective therapy. Chapter 8 addresses the issue of goal-setting. The contracting session is complete when all involved members of the problem-system necessary for implementing the plans agree to be involved in an episode of therapy. Therapeutic episodes are time limited. Common time frames are three, six or ten hourly sessions spaced at increasingly expanded intervals from between a week and three months.

The major stumbling block here is to identify goals that all members of the family can agree upon. Goals are discussed in Chapter 8.

Stage 3.2. Participating in therapy

Therapy in Positive Practice involves two main processes: focusing on behaviour and focusing on beliefs. In the first the therapist and the family work directly on breaking the cycle of interaction around the presenting problem. This often involves the family completing tasks within the session, or as homework between sessions, and reviewing the effects of these tasks on the problem. This aspect of Positive Practice, which is covered in Chapters 9 and 10, draws heavily, although not exclusively, on the structural (Colapinto, 1991), strategic (Madanes, 1991), problem-focused (Segal, 1991), solution-focused (deShazer, 1988) and behavioural traditions (Falloon, 1991) within the family therapy field.

In the second major therapeutic process, the therapist and the family aim directly to transform the belief system that underpins the pattern of interaction in which the presenting problem is embedded. If the belief system is transformed, then the pattern of interaction will change and the problem will resolve. The transformation of belief systems in Positive Practice involves the use of a variety of interviewing techniques which have evolved from the Milan Systemic Family Therapy (Campbell, Draper and Crutchley, 1991) and the emerging Post-modern tradition within the field (Gilligan and Price, 1993). These are described in parts of Chapter 10 and Chapter 11.

While much therapeutic communication within Positive Practice takes place within family therapy sessions, this is not exclusively the case. In certain circumstances therapy may occur through letter writing, individual sessions with children and network meetings involving professionals from agencies that have significant contact with the family. Letters, child-centred sessions and network meetings are discussed in Chapters 12, 14 and 15.

Stage 3.3. Troubleshooting resistance

Between contracting for therapy and agreeing to terminate the therapeutic process, many hitches will occur in most cases. For example, family members may miss appointments, not complete homework assignments, participate in therapy sessions in ways that prevent progress or revert to an individualistic formulation of the problem. On some occasions this resistance will present as a therapeutic crisis. Often therapists and other professionals in the problem-system develop countertransference reactions, in response to resistance or crises, which lead them to replicate dysfunctional patterns of interaction that occur in the families with which they work. In Positive Practice, the therapist is prepared for these and other forms of resistance and troubleshoots each resistance in a systematic way. The resistance must be described clearly, possible factors contributing to it mapped out and options for overcoming it explored. Resistance, therapeutic dilemmas, crises and countertransference are dealt with in Chapters 11 and 13.

Stage 4. Disengaging or recontracting

An episode of therapy is completed when the therapeutic plan has been implemented in its original or modified form, where whatever resistances to implementation have been dealt with, where relapse management has been discussed, and where goal attainment has been assessed.

Where therapy has been unsuccessful, as it will be in about 25% of cases (Carr, 1991a), it is vital to explore the reasons for failure with the members of the problem-system. In some instances it may be that the approach to consultation described here is an inappropriate way to reach the goals which the family have set. In such instances, the family and referring agent need to be alerted to the inappropriateness of the approach and alternatives discussed or suggested.

At the end of an episode of successful therapy (or following assessment when no therapy is offered) two routes may typically be followed. In the first, the therapist offers the family a follow-up contact in three or six months to check on progress. This may be an appointment or a telephone contact. This is a particularly useful way of keeping track of the effectiveness of the consultation process. The second route involves the therapist offering a contract for further therapy to members of the family to work on problems that remain unresolved. These may include further child-focused difficulties; personal problems that have come to light for the parents during the child focused therapy; or, more commonly, marital difficulties. Often the importance of personal therapy for parents or marital therapy become obvious during the assessment phase, but offering work in these areas is deferred until the presenting problem has been resolved.

Disengagement and recontracting is considered in Chapter 16.

CONTACT WITH THE REFERRING AGENT

At referral and disengagement, contact with the referring agent is a routine part of Positive Practice. It is also necessary to inform the referrer if the family drops out of therapy. This is particularly important where the referral was made as part of statutory child care procedures, or where the presenting problem involved the mismanagement of a dangerous medical condition such as diabetes. Whether these contacts with the referrer are verbal or written depends on the context. Where therapists are building up a referral network, brief but detailed accounts of case formulations and therapy programmes are a useful way of educating other professionals about systemic thinking and types of cases that may appropriately be referred. Where referral networks are well established, a phonecall may be more apt.

When a family reach Stage 4 and some family members wish to recontract for further therapy, the process of engagement and contracting for assessment starts once again. This is reflected in Figure 1.1 by portraying the stages of therapy as part of a feedback loop. Of course, therapist or family may exit from this loop at any time.

Ethical issues and their management are explored in Chapter 17.

Positive Practice is not only an approach to the practice of therapy, but also an approach to service development. The use of audit in the development of an overall consultation service is described in Chapter 18, along with guidelines for continuing professional development.

SUMMARY

Consultation in Positive Practice may be construed as a developmental and recursive process. The process begins with the therapist planning who to invite to the preliminary consultation and then planning an agenda. The first session opens with the therapist establishing a contract to complete an assessment, and then conducting the assessment procedures with the clients. When the assessment is complete and a formulation of the problem has been constructed, a contract for therapy is offered and goals are set. As therapy proceeds, resistance arises from various sources and the therapist and clients work to circumvent these obstacles to problem resolution. When the therapy contract is completed, the clients and the therapist may agree either to disengage or to contract for a further episode of consultation.

2

Planning Who to Invite

When a child or family are referred for consultation one of the first decisions to be made is who to invite to the first session. Do you invite the child only; the child and the mother, the child the parents and the siblings; the members of the household and the foster parents who give occasional relief care; the parents and the social worker who is contemplating care proceedings? Of course the answer is *It depends!* It depends upon who is involved with the problem and what role each of these people have with respect to the problem. To make a decision about who to invite, a systematic way of clarifying these issues is required.

Let us refer to the group of people organised around the problem at the time of referral as the problem-system (Anderson et al, 1986). Within this system certain key roles may be identified. First, there is the referring agent.

THE REFERRING AGENT

This is a crucial role, since the referring agent connects you to the child or family with the problem. Overtly, the referring agent is usually saying *Can you help this family resolve a particular problem?* Covertly the referring agent may be asking you to help him avoid some unpleasant circumstances by accepting the referral. For example, where a referrer has repeatedly failed to help a family, he may be asking for confirmation that the family is untreatable. This will help him avoid the painful conclusion that he is less than competent. Or, where a referrer is exhausted through continually monitoring a family at risk for child abuse and fears that he may become the scapegoat of an inquiry if abuse occurs, he may be asking covertly to relinquish responsibility for the case. That is, he may want to avoid being scapegoated so that he may pass the buck. If you suspect that the referring agent has a hidden agenda and this cannot be clarified by a telephone conversation, then invite the referrer to the intake interview.

THE AGENT OF SOCIAL CONTROL

The state empowers certain professionals to monitor the behaviour of family members, and to take steps to protect family members in danger of hurting themselves or other members of the family or society. Social workers, probation officers, school attendance officers, education and welfare officers and psychiatrists are some of the professionals that have this function. When you are referred a family where there is a risk of child abuse, suicidal behaviour, criminality, school non-attendance or marital violence, it is important to identify any agent of social control that may already be involved in the case. If their position with respect to the case cannot be clarified by telephone contact, then they may have some hidden agenda. Invite them to the intake interview if this is the case.

THE CUSTOMER

The customer is the person who is most concerned that you accept the referral and take action to resolve the presenting problem. Of course, there may be more than one customer in any problem-system. For example, the referring school teacher and the parents of Hugh, a child with conduct problems were all customers for change. Also, people will vary in the degree to which they are customers. For example, the teacher wanted help with managing Hugh's behavioural problems in the classroom. The parents were less concerned but nonetheless wanted the problem resolved. Finally, different customers in the same problem system will often have different reasons for wanting the referral to occur. For example, Hugh wanted the teacher to stop criticising him in front of his peers, while the teacher wanted to be able to devote more energy to teaching and less to managing the disruptive behaviour.

In some cases, a number of people will clearly not be customers for change. For example, foster parents referred by the social worker of a child in their care wanted to be left alone to manage the youngster's difficulties. He sporadically ran away from their house and they would arrange a search party to bring him back. They would then talk through the events that led to the episode and manage the situation in their own way. The foster parents were not customers for consultation. However, the social worker thought that they should have some help and so was the main customer for change in the problem-system. The customer must always be present at the intake meeting. In this case, the social worker who was the main customer and the foster parents were invited to the intake meeting with the foster child.

THE PROBLEM PERSON

When consulting to children and families, there is usually one child who is identified by the customer as the problem. The reason for referral is often framed in terms of focusing on changing some aspect of this problem person's behaviour. We have already mentioned Hugh, a lad with conduct problems. The request was to change Hugh's behaviour by eliminating these. The assessment process usually leads from an individual definition of one child's difficulties to an interactional formulation of the problem. It is useful to include the problem person in the first session so that he or she can contribute to the construction of the problem formulation which will eventually open the door to problem resolution. In some instances, inclusion of the problem person may be deferred. For example, where an infant's incessant crying is the presenting problem, it may be easier to conduct an intake meeting with the parents only. With uncooperative adolescents it may also be useful to hold the intake meeting without them. Exploring ways of recruiting them into the consultation process may be part of the agenda in such cases.

PRIMARY CAREGIVERS

The primary caregivers are those people who meet the referred child's needs on a day-to-day basis. They usually have a high level of contact with the referred child and considerable control over the physical and psychosocial environment within which the child lives. With intact traditional families, the parents are the primary caregivers. However in single parent families, reconstituted or blended families where parents are divorced and remarried or cohabiting, foster families, and situations where children are living in residential care centres special consideration needs to be given to identifying the primary caregivers. Ideally, the primary caregivers should attend the intake meeting because they have the richest store of observations of the problem child's behaviour and so are well equipped to participate in the construction of a useful formulation. They may also be the primary participants in evolving a solution because of their regular and intensive contact with the problem person.

In traditional families, one of the challenges for family therapists is to arrange clinic times flexibly so parents, particularly fathers, with daytime jobs may attend at least the intake consultation. In reconstituted families the challenge is to arrange to include the non-custodial parent in the preliminary assessment wherever possible.

THE LEGAL GUARDIANS

The legal guardians are those people legally responsible for the child's well-being. In intact traditional families, this role is usually filled by the parents. In reconstituted families, foster families and where children are in residential care, identifying the legal guardians and obtaining their consent for consultation to occur is important. The child may be a ward of court or in the care of the local County Council and formal permission may be required. The legal guardians do not have to be present at the intake meeting. They simply need to have given their consent for the consultation to occur.

CHANGE PROMOTERS

Change promoters are members of the network who may be particularly resourceful in contributing to the construction of the formulation or the evolution of the solution to the presenting problem. Siblings, extended family members, involved professionals, potentially involved professionals and self-help groups are some examples of change promoters worth keeping in mind when mapping out the problem-system of a referred case.

CHANGE PREVENTERS

Change preventers are members of the problem-system who inadvertently play a major role in maintaining the problem and preventing its resolution. For example, with the Dodwells, whose child Simon was referred because of repeated episodes of theft, the father met with the GP periodically. Both would reconstruct an individual formulation of the problem in terms that labelled Simon as intrinsically ill or criminal, and requiring either psychiatric inpatient treatment or incarceration in an institution for juvenile offenders. At other times the father would contribute to and endorse an interactional formulation of Simon's theft. But, after a visit to his GP, he would revert to an individual problem definition. In this problem-system, the GP was inadvertently a change preventer. An extended telephone conversation with the GP, followed up with a meeting, in which an interactional problem formulation was fleshed out, went some way to helping the GP move out of his role as a change preventer.

It is important to emphasise that these roles of change promoter, change preventers, and customers are useful social constructions and not characteristics of people, for example, in the way that eye colour is. These roles are designations that I have found useful in mapping out the problem-system of newly referred cases. A summary of each of the roles and the conditions under which people filling the roles should be invited to the first session, is set out in Figure 2.1.

PLANNING WHO TO INVITE FROM THE BARROW FAMILY

Caroline Barrow was referred simultaneously by both the Educational Psychologist, David Trellis and by Tom Walker, the Paediatrician. The referral letters are contained in Figures 2.2 and 2.3. After reading these, it was clear that the presenting problem had two main aspects. Caroline was reporting recurrent abdominal pain for which no organic basis could be found. She was also absent from school a great deal because of these pains.

From the information contained in the referral letters and from a telephone contact with the Educational Psychologist (described below), I listed all the involved professionals and tried to decide the role that each filled in the network. The list and the hypotheses I made about the role of network members is presented in Figure 2.4. From the Paediatrician's referring letter, I guessed that Tom Walker had no hidden agenda. He had seen Caroline in a one-off consultation, decided that her problems were primarily psychological and referred her immediately. This was common practice in our health district, and I had a good working relationship with Tom, so I could make my judgement about his role in the case with a high degree of confidence.

From David Trellis' letter I suspected that there may have been some complications in the referral process. There was the possibility that the Education and Welfare Officer (EWO) might act as an agent of social control and take the case to court because of the school non-attendance. The ongoing role of the Medical Officer and the School Nurse also needed clarification. I phoned David Trellis to get his views on these issues. He said that Phil Hutchinson had no plans for further contact with the Barrows until after they had completed the consultation process at our clinic, and that Nurse Boyd and Dr Reed were not planning further involvement either.

ROLE	DEFINITION	CONDITIONS WHERE INVITATION SHOULD BE OFFERED
Referring agent	The pivotal member of the problem system that connects the therapist, the team and the agency to the extant problem-system	Invite if the reason for referral is unclear or appears to contain some hidden agenda
Agent of Social Control	Representatives of the state, statutorily empowered to intervene in clients' lives without consent for the common good. Social workers, probation officers and psychiatrists often fill this role	Invite if the reason for referral is unclear or appears to contain some hidden agenda
Customer	Any system member that has an investment in the problem being resolved. There may be more than one customer	Always invite the main customer
Problem Person	The person identified by the referrer or the customer as the individual requiring help	Only exclude the problem person if he or she is very unwilling to come (e.g. adolescent), or if the customer would find it very difficult to talk about the problem with the problem person present (e.g. infant)
Primary Caregivers	Usually the mother and father, but may be a sibling or foster parents	Include as many of these as possible in the first session, particularly fathers and non-custodial parents
Legal Guardians	Usually the parents but may be the local authority (represented by a social worker) when children are in care	They need not attend the first session but their consent to proceed with the consultation is essential
Change Promoters	Those who have resources to contribute to resolving the presenting problems and who are available to do so	Need not be included in first session but may be included in later sessions
Change Preventers	Those who prevent problem resolution and maintain homeostasis	Need not be included in the first session but may be included in later sessions

Figure 2.1.   Who to invite to the first session

I suspected that Mr and Mrs Barrow would view the EWO as a threat and would want to avoid court involvement and therefore accept a preliminary appointment for themselves and their children. However, one of our main concerns was that if the Barrows viewed us as aligned with the EWO, they would withdraw from treatment because they would see us as coercive. We planned to clarify our neutrality early on in the consultation process.

Queen Mary Hospital
Market Town
Norfolk
9.2.90

Dr A. Carr
The Child & Family Centre
Market Town
Norfolk

Re: Caroline Barrow (DOB 2.2.76), 14 Telltale Close, Newtown.

Dear Alan:

The casualty officer asked me to take look at this girl today. She came in complaining of abdominal pain. Appendicitis was expected but not confirmed. Indeed the pain resolved itself before I had a chance to examine her.

The history is as follows. These recurrent abdominal pains have been present for 6 months. In the past few weeks they have been accompanied by headaches and occasionally nausea and vomiting. The symptoms are worst in the mornings. The girl has missed a lot of school over the past couple of terms.

I spoke to the GP, Dr Wilson, on the phone. He has seen the girl quite frequently over the past year although not so much this past month or two. Caroline's mother appears to be very concerned and has attended the surgery regularly with her daughter.

It's a puzzling case. Routine examination and investigations are all negative. I suspect this may be a hysterical or psychosomatic condition.

Please assess and advise.

Yours sincerely

Dr Tom Walker
Consultant Paediatrician

Figure 2.2.   The Paediatrician's referral letter

School Psychological Service
Market Town
Norfolk
7.2.90

Dr A. Carr
The Child & Family Centre
Market Town
Norfolk

Re: Caroline Barrow (DOB 2.2.76), 14 Telltale Close, Newtown.
Pupil at Ringwood High School, Market Town

Dear Alan:

This girl has been causing a lot of concern at Ringwood recently. The Education and Welfare officer, Phil Hutchinson, has been involved because of Caroline's poor school attendance. The school nurse, Nurse Boyd, and the Clinical Medical Officer, Dr Reed have both seen her from time to time for headaches and cramps. However, my impression is that they have both given her a clean bill of health.

We have recently reached an impasse. Phil (the EWO) advised the parents to return Caroline to school in the light of the CMO's opinion that the girl was medically fit. Mr and Mrs Barrow didn't co-operate. I was asked to do a home visit. My impression is that it is a simple case of school refusal. I know that you have an interest in this area, hence the referral.

(Also, as you know, because of the re-organization, I will not be responsible for Ringwood after next month and no-one has been appointed to fill my post.)

Many thanks for accepting this referral.

David Trellis
Educational Psychologist

Figure 2.3.   The Educational Psychologist's referral letter

Person	Position	Main Role
Dr Tom Walker	Paediatrician	Referrer
David Trellis	Educational Psychologist	Referrer
Caroline Barrow	Daughter	Problem Person
Mrs Barrow	Mother	Primary Caregiver Legal Guardian Main Customer
Mr Barrow	Father	Primary Caregiver Legal Guardian
Miss Boyd	School Nurse	Possible Change Promoter
Dr Reed	Clinical Medical Officer	Possible Change Promoter
Dr Wilson	GP	Possible Change Promoter

Figure 2.4. Hypotheses about roles of members in the Barrow's problem system

From the Paediatrician's letter I suspected that Mrs Barrow was the main customer. He pointed out that she regularly attended the GP with her daughter. I decided that it would be sufficient to invite Caroline and her parents, along with any other members of the household to the first session. A letter was therefore sent inviting the Barrow family for a preliminary consultation.

We will return to the Barrow case in Chapter 3 to explore the preliminary formulation that guided the lines of questioning followed in the first interview. Before moving on to that, let us first consider some common difficulties that occur when errors are made in deciding who to invite to the intake session, or when those invited do not turn up.

ENGAGEMENT MISTAKES

Engagement is the first and most critical aspect of the consultation process (Carr, 1990a). If mistakes are made here, then the chances of therapy being successful are greatly reduced. In many cases where therapy reaches an impasse, where progress is negligible, or where dropout occurs, some type of engagement difficulty may be identified (Coleman, 1985). Because these are rarely pinpointed, we are often mystified or angered by such therapeutic failures.

Selecting those members of the problem-system who will be most effective in helping to resolve the presenting problem is the key to avoiding engagement difficulties. However, this selection process is fraught with difficulties. There are many pitfalls along the way. Most stem from assumptions and beliefs that are held by the therapist. Some of these are presented here, along with suggestions for dealing with these engagement mistakes, should you inadvertently find yourself making them.

1. **Assuming that the nuclear family of the problem person is the unit of treatment and failing to take account of other network members**

Often key members of the problem-system lie outside the nuclear family. This group may include members of extended family, step-family, adoptive-family and foster-family. It may include peers and colleagues from work settings, and members of religious, recreational and other community-based organisations. It may also include a variety of statutory and non-statutory professionals such as physicians, social workers, probation officers, health visitors, dieticians etc. The solution to this engagement problem is to be careful not to draw an artificial boundary around the nuclear family when mapping out the roles that those involved play in the problem-system.

2. **Assuming that the person legally responsible for the problem person is the customer, when the referring agent is customer**

This mistake usually occurs in cases where conduct problems are the central concern (e.g. Carl and Jurkovic, 1983). A school principal referred a boy and his family for therapy, via the GP, because of the boy's disruptive behaviour in school. The family did not attend the intake interview. A phone call to the GP revealed that the parents felt antagonistic towards the school and were ambivalent about our unit, which they viewed as aligned with the school. Here, the school was the customer.

To avoid this error it is useful to clarify by phone if the referring agent is the customer. If this is the case, the referring agent may be asked to be responsible for the family's attendance at the intake interview and to attend this meeting themselves. The focus of such meetings is to help the person legally responsible for the problem-person and the referring agent clarify the pros and cons of the problem person, and the person legally responsible for the problem person in committing themselves to a therapeutic contract.

3. **Assuming that the problem person's emotionally attached caregiver is the customer when the referring agent is the customer**

This mistake may occur in cases where attachment difficulties between parents and children are the central presenting problem.

A social worker referred a young single mother and her two-year-old daughter for therapy. The social worker described the mother and child as having *poor bonding*. The mother often left the child to cry for periods of up to an hour and frequently felt as if the baby were trying intentionally to annoy her. The mother said that she wanted help with finding a way to deal with her child's crying. She also agreed to explore ways in which she could increase the social support available to her as an isolated single parent. However, her attendance at therapy was erratic and she rarely completed homework assignments. I invited her and the referring social worker to a meeting to explore reasons for the therapeutic failure. It transpired that the mother believed that the social worker had decided to take the child into care. The referral had been an attempt on the social worker's part, she believed, to prove that she could not be helped. No matter how hard she tried to benefit from the therapy, she believed that ultimately the social worker would take her baby into care. Therefore, she put little effort into the venture. She was not the customer. Rather, the customer in this case was the social worker.

Subsequently, the social worker attended a series of sessions in which she stated explicitly, in behavioural terms, the expectations held by her department of competent parents. This convinced the mother that her parenting was indeed competent. I then offered a contract to the mother for therapy that would focus on *enriching* her relationship with her child, since the social worker's criteria had demonstrated that remedial therapy was not required.

4. Assuming that the referring agent has a positive alliance with all family members

If the referring agent has a very strong alliance with one or two members of the overall problem-system and neutral or negative alliances with others, the therapist may be sucked into a particular role in the family drama which renders her impotent. Usually this role is one that was previously occupied by the referring agent. Selvini Palazzoli (1980b) and her colleagues have described this problem in cases where the referring agent is a close friend of one family member. Physicians (either GPs or specialists) who have been treating one family member for years, counsellors who are very supportive of the mother in the family, and social workers who act as a go-between with the patient and the parents, are the three main categories of referring agent identified by the Milan group in their study of this problem. The referring agent feels disqualified and trapped. In the final stage, the referral is made when the referring agent has become exasperated.

The Milan group noted that when they accepted referrals like these without including the referring agent in the initial meetings, or at least without discussing the family's relationship with the referring agent, therapy was ineffective. The team slipped into fulfilling the same function as the referring agent. They dealt with this problem by prescribing continued contact with the referring agent and positively connoting all that he or she had done.

Selvini Palazzoli (1985) has also described the difficulties that arise in cases where a prestigious sibling of the problem-person is the referring agent. Usually the sibling has a close relationship with one parent and holds a privileged and powerful position within the family. The demands of new relationships outside the family, however, make the sibling feel tied down. He sees family therapy as a way of liberating himself from his exacting role. There is also the possibility that the prestigious referring sibling has begun to grow envious of the love and attention which the problem sibling commands. The key to the Milan group's approach has been to avoid slipping into the referring sibling's shoes by attempting to do therapy with the remainder of the family.

Selvini Palazzoli (1985) describes how she and the Milan team first offered a family referred by a sibling an assessment, to see if they were suitable for family therapy. During the assessment, the pattern of interaction which surrounded the problem person and included the parents, the siblings and the referring sibling was established. At the conclusion of the assessment, the therapist then described this pattern, positively connoting the role of problem person in creating a prestigious position within the family for the referring sibling to occupy. She then said that family therapy was not indicated, since it would lead to improvement in the problem person, which would destroy the privileged position of the referring person in the family and lead to him becoming depressed. The problem daughter spontaneously improved and the referring sibling left home to live in his own apartment.

5. Failing to identify system members that promote stuckness

This error can occur when the therapist assumes that the nuclear family is the unit of treatment, but where the boundaries of the nuclear family are fairly diffuse and family members rely on close ties with members of their extended family for carrying out the tasks of day-to-day living.

A single parent of borderline intelligence and her nine-year-old son, who had mainly home-based conduct problems, were referred by the GP. An assessment showed that when the mother asked the boy to do something to which he objected, he would often throw a tantrum. The mother managed these tantrums inconsistently. It appeared that the tantrums continued because most of the time they got him what he wanted. It seemed that the mother's inconsistency persisted because she did not know what else to do. It was not related to emotional exhaustion since the mother was well supported emotionally, both by her sister who lived locally and by members of her church.

At the conclusion of the first session the mother and son agreed to carry out two homework tasks. The first involved the mother spending half an hour a day with her son doing painting, his favourite activity. They understood that this regular period of positive interaction was to rebuild the positive side of their relationship which had become tainted with bitterness. The second task involved the boy going to *time-out* under his mother's supervision whenever he lost his temper, so that he could learn how to control it himself.

The mother and son consistently executed the temper control task incorrectly. The mother would let the boy out of his bedroom immediately he began swearing and cursing. Careful interviewing revealed that she abhorred swearing because of her religious beliefs. She would rather her boy got his own way than be eternally damned for swearing—and she was certain that her vicar would take the same view. Thus the vicar (and possibly God) were system members promoting stuckness whom I had failed to identify.

I made arrangements to meet the vicar and, after some discussion about the rationale behind the tasks, he convinced the mother to go along with the homework assignments. In the long run, he said, they would help her son avoid sin and keep to the path of righteousness.

System members who promote stuckness may reside not only out in the wider community but also in the memories of members of the nuclear family. When therapists focus on current patterns of interaction without reference to past relationships, and where introjects or ghosts are a significant part of the family drama, therapists may fail to identify these system members. These stuckness-promoting-system-members may be estranged or deceased and so physically absent from the problem-system. However, as introjects or ghosts, they continue to have a powerful constraining influence on the search for a workable solution to the presenting problem. Usually the member of the problem-system influenced by the ghost will require a forum within which to complete unfinished business.

In an initial interview with the mother of a thirteen-year-old-girl referred because of her aggressive and defiant conduct, it emerged that the girl's problem behaviour only occurred in specific circumstances. When mother, stepfather and daughter were together and stepfather showed more interest in the girl than in his wife, or where mother believed that this scenario was imminent, mother and daughter would fight. So as to establish how the presenting problem would have been dealt with in the mother's family of origin, I asked the mother how *her* mother would have shared her father.

The mother became distressed in response to this enquiry. It emerged that at the age of thirteen she had become involved in an incestuous relationship with her father and feared that her daughter and husband might be about to replicate this pattern. The deceased grandfather in the family was a ghost who promoted stuckness.

The parents of the thirteen-year-old were seen on a number of occasions without their daughter so that the mother could address the unfinished business with her incestuous deceased father. Concurrent family work focusing on straightforward parent-adolescent negotiation progressed without any major impasses.

6. Failing to distinguish the role of therapist from the role of agent of social control

An agency may have statutory functions but may also offer a therapeutic service. This is true of departments of social services, probation, police, psychiatry and education. A social services department, for example, is empowered by the state to protect children by requesting that a court remove them from the custody of their parents. The department may also offer a family therapy service, but if a worker confuses these two functions, good therapy will not be offered.

When workers exercise statutory powers, they act as social control agents for the state. They define and control the limits of an individual's or family's liberty. Inevitably, the client whose freedom has been limited through the exercise of statutory power will feel antagonistic towards the statutory worker. For these two individuals then to attempt to develop a therapeutic alliance is difficult. It requires the client to distinguish between the *worker as therapist* from the *worker as agent of social control*. Maintaining this distinction requires a constant input of energy from both parties over and above that necessary for therapy. If the distinction is not maintained, the clients may go through the motions of therapy so as to appease their *statutory controller*, or the client may drop out of therapy.

There is also a danger of this process occurring even when the statutory worker and the therapist are separate individuals. This is well illustrated by the example given earlier where a mother and child were referred to me by a social worker because of their attachment difficulties. Although I was in a different agency from the referring social worker, and no threat of statutory action had been made, the client still viewed both me and the referring agent as agents of social control.

In cases where statutory action has been taken or is likely to occur and therapy is offered, the therapist must devise a set of strategies to convince the client that the therapy is distinct from the social control. One useful arrangement is for the statutory worker to set clearly defined and observable criteria which must be met before the statutory limits which have been placed on the client's freedom may be wholly or partially withdrawn. The worker may then refer the case to a therapist, requesting that the client be offered a contract for therapy which involves searching for ways to meet the criteria posed by the statutory worker. The statutory worker may then periodically assess therapeutic progress according to the predefined criteria (Crowther et al, 1990).

7. Failing to take account of the image projected by the agency to prospective clients

The image the agency projects will affect engagement and the therapy process. For example, clients may view probation offices and social work departments as being staffed by social control agents. Hospitals and private therapeutic institutes may be viewed as the workplaces of helpful professionals. Family therapy was originally developed in the latter type of settings. However, a sizeable number of practitioners now practice within the former types of agencies.

In taking family therapy lock, stock and barrel as practised in one agency context, and attempting to replicate this in another without taking account of how the agency is perceived by the client group, may lead to engagement problems. For example, Howe (1989) found that clients attending a social services staffed family therapy agency had difficulty participating in family therapy and experiencing benefit from the live supervision which was available to the therapist. In fact the live supervision provided by the team via close circuit television was one of the key factors leading to the clients' sense of powerlessness. These difficulties occurred, in part, because the therapist and team assumed that their clients were well informed customers who wanted the form of intervention being offered. Howe's study suggests that many of the clients were frightened to voice their opinions and none asked to be referred to another practitioner. Howe's study points to the importance of redressing the perceived imbalance of power for clients who seek therapeutic services from statutory agencies through providing a brief educational induction programme prior to therapy. Such a programme should highlight the details of how the therapeutic process will proceed, the voluntary nature of the treatment contract and the other locally available treatment options (Pimpernell and Treacher, 1990). If we are to be truly systemic in our outlook we must include therapist, team and agency in our initial formulations. We must make hypotheses about how we are perceived by our clients, test these out and take steps to correct misapprehensions. This is precisely the course of action taken by the team, although regrettably this information was omitted from Howe's book (*Reflection*, 1989).

SUMMARY

The decision about who to invite to the first consultation session should be based upon an analysis of the roles played by the members of the problem-system. These roles include the referring agent, customer, the problem person, those legally responsible for the problem person, the primary caregivers, system members who promote stuckness and system members who promote change. The customer must be present at the intake meeting and the legal guardian of the referred child must have given consent for the referral to occur. Ideally, the problem person and the primary caretakers should also be present. With infants or reluctant adolescents, it may be more productive to hold the first session without the problem person. Where an agent of social control is involved, or potentially involved, they should also be present for the intake meeting. Referring agents should be contacted or included in the first session if there appears to be a hidden agenda.

Engagement mistakes can lead to therapeutic failure. Some of these mistakes occur because the most useful constellation of members from the problem system were not invited to the first session. This in turn may have been due to certain beliefs, attitudes and assumptions on the therapists part. Common engagement mistakes include the following:

1. Assuming that the nuclear family of the problem person is the unit of measurement and failing to take account of other network members.
2. Assuming that the person legally responsible for the problem person is the customer, when the referring agent is the customer.
3. Assuming that the problem person's emotionally attached caregiver is the customer, when the referring agent is the customer.
4. Assuming that the referring agent has a positive alliance with all family members.
5. Failing to Identify system members that promote stuckness.
6. Failing to distinguish the role of therapist from the role of agent of social control.
7. Failing to take account of the image projected by the agency to prospective clients.

EXERCISE 2.1.

Work in pairs.

Read the following referral letter alone or in teams of between 2 and 4 members. Then decide what role each person plays in the problem system using Table 2. 1. as a framework. Finally decide who to invite to the first session.

Referral Letter

The Surgery
Any Town

3.5.93

Dear Colleague

Re: Dawn Rooney, (DOB 3.2. 88). Seaview Terrace, Oldsville.

Dawn has been a regular attender at the surgery with her mother over the past year. She is a fine healthy young girl but is alternatively very clingy and very disobedient. She is an only child.

The problems are worst after those weekends when she visits with her father. (The parents, who cohabited for Dawn's first year of life, are separated).

The Grandmother, also a patient of mine, cares for Dawn when Rose (Ms Rooney) is at work. She says that the girl is fine at her house and blames the problems on her daughter's free and easy approach to discipline.

Over the past year things have deteriorated steadily to a point where, last week, Dawn nearly fell out of her bedroom window. Rose is distraught. The befriender (Nancy Byrne) who has been visiting to offer support on a fortnightly basis is very frustrated with the case.

I think we really need you to take a close look at this one and see how Dawn may be helped to overcome her difficulties.

Thank you for your help

Yours sincerely

Dr Frank Walsh
Family Doctor

3

Planning What to Ask

In Positive Practice the agenda for the first meeting is based on three considerations. First, the therapist must deal with any possible engagement difficulties by clarifying the position of the therapist in relation to other members of the problem-system. Usually this involves explaining how the referral occurred and stating that the therapist is neutral with respect to other members of the problem-system. Second, the therapist must take account of the developmental nature of the consultation process by establishing a contract for assessment at the outset. Third, the therapist must facilitate the construction of a useful problem formulation that will point to a feasible solution. In Positive Practice the three column model is used as a framework for constructing problem formulations (Carr, 1990b). This model will be described in detail below.

When planning lines of inquiry to pursue during the first session to help construct a useful formulation, the three column model is used to systematise the therapist's hunches and hypotheses. Hunches and hypotheses will usually be based on the therapist's experience with similar cases, her knowledge of the relevant literature and other life experiences. The therapist uses the three column model to draw up a preliminary formulation, and then plans to ask the family about the presenting problem, their histories, their beliefs and their typical ways of living together in a focused way guided by the preliminary formulation. In Positive Practice, the therapist never simply takes a developmental history or draws up a problem list. Always historical or problem based inquiries are made in a focused way with a view to testing a hypothesis which will allow the elaboration of some aspect of the formulation.

In planning what to ask the Barrow family in the first session, I began by clarifying my own hunches and constructing a preliminary formulation to guide my lines of questioning.

DEVELOPMENT OF A PRELIMINARY FORMULATION FOR THE BARROW FAMILY

My preliminary hunch was that Caroline and her mother were involved in a relationship characterised by separation anxiety on both of their parts, which manifested itself through Caroline experiencing abdominal pain and through the mother and daughter avoiding separation. This in turn led to school avoidance. We further hypothesised that some set of family or work-based circumstances prevented the father from intervening in this anxiety-ridden relationship. Finally, we suspected that the mother and father held beliefs rooted in some remote or recent stressful life events within the family which prevented them from dealing with the separation anxiety problem and Caroline's related abdominal pain and school refusal. There was also the possibility that Caroline had a history of gastric complaints and so was vulnerable to developing abdominal pain. The anxiety may have been exacerbated by the lack of explicit recognition given to it by virtually all of the involved professionals. The involved physicians and nurses, in the absence of evidence of organic pathology, were construing the abdominal pain as either *not real* or *not important*. The Education and Welfare Officer, armed with this medical information was interpreting Caroline's school refusal as truancy, and threatening to use his statutory power to bring this truancy to the attention of the courts. A diagram of this preliminary formulation, in three column format, is presented in Figure 3.1. Our

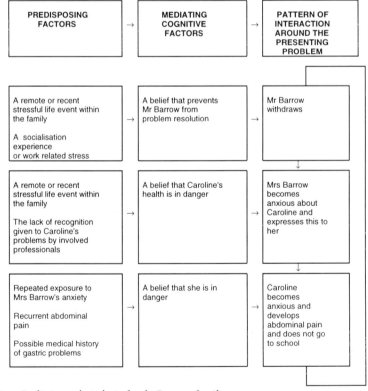

Figure 3.1.   Preliminary hypothesis for the Barrow family

formulation was based on the information in the referral letters, and was informed by available research on school-refusal (e.g. Hersov, 1985), and by our experience with a series of these cases which we had seen over a three year period. Let us turn now to an exploration of the three column model and examine in more detail how it was used to organise our hunches about the Barrow case, and how it may be used with other cases.

THE THREE COLUMN MODEL FOR CONSTRUCTING HYPOTHESES

In the right hand column of this model, the suspected pattern of interaction containing the symptom or presenting problem in which the problem person and members of the problem-system are caught up, is set out. In the left hand column, factors which it is suspected predispose participants in this cycle to persist in this repetitive sequence of interaction is noted. In the central column, suspected beliefs or styles of information processing which mediate the influence of predisposing factors on the present cycle of activity are listed.

Patterns of Interaction

The hypothesised pattern of interaction in the right hand column will provide a basis for inquiring about specific events that trigger an episode of the presenting problem, the reactions of members of the problem-system to the problem when it is occurring and the way the problem person and other members of the problem-system conclude each episode. With the Barrow family, a line of questioning inquiring about what Mr and Mrs Barrow did before, during and after an episode of Caroline's abdominal pain was planned. Inquiries about the cycle of interaction around the symptom would throw light on how members of the system try to solve the presenting problem and also what the costs and benefits of being involved in an episode are for family members.

We hoped that the Barrow's answers to our questions about an episode of the problem would give us clues to their ineffectual problem-solving strategies and how these attempts at solving the problem might in fact be reinforcing or maintaining it. This idea, that often people's solutions to a little problem generate a bigger problem is the cornerstone of the model of family therapy developed by the Palo Alto group (Segal, 1991). The idea is well captured by their catchphrase *The solution is the problem.*

Gregory Bateson's classification of dyadic relationships as symmetrical or complimentary would also inform our inquiries about the interactional pattern related to the symptom (Bateson, 1973). Where parents are caring for a sick child and a complimentary relationship develops, the more the parent tends to the child, the more care the child appears to require. That is, in a complimentary relationship, one person adopts a *one-up* position while the other adopts a *one-down* position. As the relationship evolves, the positions become more entrenched. In symmetrical relationships, both people try to adopt a *one-up* position. Parents and children who become involved in symmetrical relationships develop escalating patterns of antagonistic interaction.

Symmetrical relationships between parents and children with conduct problems have been described in detail by Gerry Patterson (1982), a behavioural family therapist. He has shown how parents and children often become embroiled in reciprocal escalating patterns of antagonistic interaction which culminate in the child and parent both withdrawing from mutual interaction. This withdrawal leads both parent and child to experience relief. This experience of relief is reinforcing for both the parent and the child. Thus, the escalating antagonistic behaviour of both parent and child is more likely to happen in the future.

Dyadic relationships, and indeed entire family patterns of relationships, may be characterized by emotional closeness or enmeshment on the one hand or emotional distance or disengagement on the other. Structural family therapists, such as Salvador Minuchin, were among the first to highlight that parent-child relationships character-ized by either extreme enmeshment or disengagement are often associated with problems (Colapinto, 1991). In our interview with the Barrows, our tracking of the pattern of interaction around the symptom would be informed by this construct.

Triadic (and multi-member) relationships within families are usefully described with reference to the constructs of boundaries, hierarchy, coalition and triangulation. These constructs are drawn largely from the structural and strategic schools of family therapy (Colapinto, 1991; Madanes, 1991). Boundaries are conceptual ring-fences that separate family factions or subsystems. For example, in families with teenagers there is usually a clear, yet permeable, boundary between the parents on the one hand and the children on the other. This boundary may be marked by the parents creating opportu-nities to spend time together away from the children. In families where boundaries are too diffuse, parents and children may be involved in enmeshed relationships. In families where boundaries are too rigid, relationships may be disengaged. Patterns of interaction that subserve diffuse or rigid boundaries are often associated with problem behaviour.

Hierarchy refers to the power structure within a family. It may be clear who has the decision making power within a family or there may be confusion about the family hierarchy. Haley (1967) has named one common family pattern where the hierarchy is confused, the pathological triangle. This is where it is overtly accepted that both parents share decision making power but where one parent (often the mother) is involved in a covert cross-generational coalition with a child.

Triangulation refers to patterns of interaction where a third person, usually a child, adopts a go-between or peace-making role which diffuses the conflict between two other family members, usually the parents. The typical scenario is where the parents become involved in a symmetrically escalating argument, and at a certain point the child engages in problem behaviour such as reporting a headache or misbehaving. The child's behaviour temporarily diffuses the parental conflict but does not solve it. Rigid patterns of triangulation often maintain symptomatic behaviour in children. With the Barrows, the notions of the pathological triangle and triangulation would inform our inquiries about the pattern of interaction around the symptom.

A system for describing and classifying patterns of interaction around presenting problems is currently being developed by Karl Tomm (1991). He refers to such patterns as Pathologizing Interpersonal Patterns (PIPs). For example, with conduct problems a common PIP is

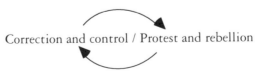

Correction and control / Protest and rebellion

With depression a common PIP is

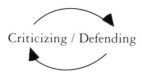

Criticizing / Defending

These PIPs are the material which is usually included in the right hand column of the three column formulation model. It is worth mentioning that PIPs are only one aspect of Tomm's classification of interpersonal patterns of interaction. For each PIP, there is an associated healing interpersonal pattern (HIP) and families trapped in PIPs may move towards HIPs by engaging in transforming interpersonal patterns (TIPs). Relapses occur because of Slips. These are stressful events which trigger the regression from HIPs to PIPs.

Predisposing Factors

Possible predisposing factors are noted in the left hand column of the model. These are factors that predispose family members to become repeatedly involved in the pattern of interaction surrounding the presenting problem. Five main classes of predisposing factors are worth noting. However, only some of these classes are relevant to the Barrow case. Remote and recent stressful life events within the family constitute the first subcategory of predisposing factors. Poor maternal bonding, early multiplacement experience, loss of a parent in childhood and a personal history of neglect or abuse are examples of remote stressful life events (Wolkind and Rutter, 1985). Financial difficulties or changes in family composition are common recent stressful life events (McCubbin and Patterson, 1991). With the Barrow family we planned to ask about events in the mother's life that may have predisposed her to being anxious about her daughter's health, and in the father's life that may have prevented him from taking a more active role in helping his wife.

The second subcategory of predisposing factors includes involvement with other social systems which make stressful demands upon the individual, such as school, work or unsympathetic mental health agencies (Walker, 1985). In the Barrow's case we planned to inquire in detail about the mother's dealings with all of the involved professionals and agencies. We also planned to inquire about the demands made upon the father by his work commitments, and to assess the degree to which this led him to adopt a peripheral role (Minuchin, 1974).

Debilitating somatic states and vulnerabilities are contained in the third subcategory. Of relevance here was our plan to inquire about Caroline's history of stomach complaints. She may have had a vulnerability to gastric difficulties. Relevant temperamental characteristics or personality traits are included in the fourth subcategory (Rutter, 1987). The final subcategory includes functional vulnerabilities which have a genetic basis, such as those which have been documented for certain types of learning disabilities and certain psychoses (McGuffin and Gottesman, 1985). We did not make explicit plans in the Barrow case to inquire about either of these sets of factors in the intake interview, since there were no grounds to suspect that these factors were present.

PREDISPOSING FACTORS	MEDIATING COGNITIVE FACTORS	PATTERN OF INTERACTION AROUND THE PRESENTING PROBLEM

Remote stressful life events
 	
Recent stressful life events
 	
Membership of stressful social systems
 	
Debilitating somatic states
 	
Temperament and personality traits
 	
Genetic vulnerabilities
	Beliefs systems
	
	Beliefs about problems and solutions relevant to the presenting problem
	
	Beliefs about parenting and family relationships
	
	Styles of information processing
	
	Attributional style
	  Internal, global, stable
	  attributions for
	  problem behaviour
	
	Cognitive distortions
	  Maximising negatives
	  Minimising positives
	
	Defence mechanisms
	  Denial
	  Displacement
	  Reaction formation
	  Rationalisation
		The problem person's symptoms and problem behaviour
		
		The sequence of events that typically precede and follow an episode of the symptoms or problem behaviour
		
		The feelings and emotions that accompany these behaviours, particularly positive feelings or payoffs
		
		Symmetrical and complimentary behavioural patterns.
		
		Enmeshed and disengaged behavioural patterns
		
		Pathological triangles and triangulation

Figure 3.2.   Three column formulation model

Mediating Cognitive Factors: Belief Systems

Predisposing factors in the first column of the three column model are linked to the pattern of interaction around the symptom in the third column by mediating cognitive factors. There are two important categories of mediating cognitive factors: belief systems and styles of information processing (including defence mechanisms).

Some predisposing factors are linked to the way in which individuals participate in the pattern of interaction around the symptom by belief systems. Often these belief systems are organised sets of premises, assumptions, attitudes and expectations which individuals hold about themselves and others which have implications for the way in which they try to solve the presenting problem. These belief systems are often conscious and are almost always accessible to consciousness. They include elements which range in magnitude and entrenchment from, for example, the automatic thoughts described by cognitive therapists (Beck and Weishaar, 1989), to the scripts described by transactional analysts (Dusay et al, 1989) and family myths referred to by many family therapists (Byng-Hall, 1988). These beliefs, scripts and myths may be hierarchically organized (Cronen and Pearse, 1985). At each level, certain central organizing themes or core-constructs may be identified (Kelly, 1955). In the Barrow case, on the basis of the central column of the hypothesis, we planned to inquire about the father's beliefs about involvement in parenting generally and specifically his beliefs about how best to conceptualise Caroline's difficulties. We planned to inquire about the mother's beliefs about the danger her daughter's health was in and how this danger might be resolved. We also planned to ask Caroline how she construed the dangerousness of her situation. In each of these lines of inquiry we hoped to link predisposing factors, via current belief systems about problems and solutions of the type the family faced, to their involvement in the current pattern of interaction around Caroline's symptoms.

Mediating Cognitive Factors: Styles of Information Processing and Defence Mechanisms

The effects of predisposing factors on participation in the pattern of interaction around the symptom may be mediated not only by belief systems but also by styles of information-processing. Stressful early life events predispose individuals to processing information in peculiar ways when faced with stressful events that are reminiscent of these in later life.

For example, a father whose mother was hospitalised for a long period while he was a child may deny or minimise symptoms of illness in his wife or children in adulthood. This peculiar way of perceiving his wife's or child's state of health may be an unconscious attempt on his part to avoid a repetition of the painful experience of abandonment which he had felt as a child. These peculiar styles of information processing may lock the individual into the pattern of interaction surrounding the symptom. Usually, there is some payoff or gain for the person using the unusual style of information processing. In the example just given the payoff for the father is the avoidance of psychological pain associated with being abandoned by an ill loved one.

Defence mechanisms described by psychodynamic therapists (Ursano and Hales, 1986), distortions described by cognitive therapists (Beck and Weishaar, 1989), and various attributional processes described by functional family therapists (Barton and Alexander, 1981), are examples of styles of information processing. These processes are largely unconscious. They are observed by the therapist rather than reported by the clients. A number of these styles of information processing deserve mention because they are so commonly seen in family work.

Parents attributing children's problem behaviour or symptoms to internal, stable, global factors rather than to external, temporary, specific factors is one of the most common problematic information processing styles with which family therapists have to deal. Parents say *My child is always sick or sad or bad* rather than *In this situation, now, my child feels sick or sad or like misbehaving.* This attributional style is often associated with the two defence mechanisms: projection and splitting. With projection, the parent directs anger and disapproval at the child because the child embodies some characteristic that the parent dislikes about him or herself, such as vulnerability or aggression. With splitting, the parent can only construe the child as either good or bad. The parent has difficulty integrating positive and negative aspects of the child into a coherent picture.

A second set of information processing problems include magnifying problems, minimising strengths and catastrophizing about the future. Here the parents say *This is a terrible problem. The signs of hope we have seen are only flashes in the pan. Things will only get worse.* This cognitive style is common when parents are depressed and has been extensively described by Beck and other cognitive therapists (Beck and Weishaar, 1989).

A third information processing difficulty is that of denial. For example, a father may refuse to acknowledge the existence of a child's difficulty. A fourth information processing style is the defence mechanism: displacement. Typically, anger that one parent has towards another is directed at a child. Displacement is the defence mechanism that underpins scapegoating and detouring marital conflict through a child. These are patterns that have been well described by structural family therapists (Colapinto, 1991). The defence mechanism, reaction formation, is a fifth problematic information processing style. For example, a parent may be angry at a child for soiling itself and go overboard to treat it well in that situation, but then be unjustifiably angry or critical the next day when the child spills a glass of water. A sixth information processing style is the defence mechanism: rationalisation. Here, parents do something which they believe is unacceptable, such as beating a child, and then they convince themselves that this was what they intended by arguing that it will help the child to develop a strong character.

In the Barrow case we suspected that the father may have been denying the existence of a problem, and so would have been less accepting of a therapeutic contract than would his wife. Dealing with this by joining with the father early in the consultation process was part of the plan for the intake interview.

SUMMARY OF THE INTAKE INTERVIEW PLAN

Let us summarise the interview plan for the Barrow family. The core of this plan is based on lines of questioning derived from the preliminary three column formulation. Other aspects of the interview plan are based on a consideration of possible engagement difficulties discussed in Chapter 2. Finally, some elements of the interview plan are founded on the developmental model which underpins the Positive Practice approach to consultation described in Chapter 1.

Contracting

1. Establish a good working relationship with Mr Barrow early in the interview (because of probable problem denial).
2. Engage the family by describing the route of referral, defining the neutral position of the clinic with respect to the referral and checking that all family members were customers for change.
3. Offer a contract for assessment.

Assessment

4. Identify the precipitating event. Why now?
5. Inquire about the pattern of interaction around the problem and exceptional circumstances where it does not occur.

6. Inquire about problem-solution beliefs that underpin this pattern.
7. Observe information processing styles (father's possible denial of the problem).
8. Inquire about predisposing factors including the mother's experiences related to health, and the father's involvement at work. Complete a genogram and family history here.
9. Take a break.

Contract for treatment

10. Integrate information into provisional formulation and develop a monitoring task.
11. Present provisional formulation to the family.
12. Define the problem as solvable.
13. Offer a contract for further consultation and the next appointment time.
14. Give a monitoring homework.

COMMENTS ON THE THREE COLUMN MODEL

The model provides a way for therapists to integrate lineal and circular ways of construing presenting problems. In the right hand column, the pattern of interaction which surrounds the presenting problem is described. This is a circular description of the problem. However, the actions of each person in this pattern of interaction are linked in a lineal way to predisposing factors in the first column via mediating cognitive factors in the second column.

The model is based on the notion that people with behavioural problems and members of their social networks become embroiled in vicious cycles of problems and inappropriate solutions. Such cycles of interaction maintain presenting problems. Participants fail to break out of such cycles because certain beliefs or ways of processing information based on personal or historical factors inhibit them from altering their roles in these stereotyped patterns of interaction.

A major problem that clinicians face in family consultation is information overload. Distressed families present clinicians with a wealth of information in a single interview. The clinician's task is to attend to essential aspects of this selectively so as to co-construct a formulation of the problem that will open up feasible options for problem-resolution. A central problem for the therapist and the family is distinguishing the essential from the incidental. Research and theory in the family therapy field has become so complex that novices who are trying to use their reading to inform their practice become overwhelmed by the amount of factors that the literature suggests they should be selectively attending to. The three column model provides a framework for simplifying and systematising hypotheses, and subsequently for integrating information relevant to these into a formulation.

The three column model suggests important lines of inquiry that the clinician should follow. The presenting problem is first clarified. Then the pattern of interaction around it is established. The beliefs that constrain family members within this cycle are then explored. This is followed by questions about predisposing factors.

The information given about the pattern of interaction around the presenting problem will throw light on key system members involved in problem maintenance. This may suggest system members that need to be included in future consultations or, if this is not feasible, they at least need to be taken account of in planning interventions. The pattern of interaction around the problem will also throw important light on previously tried ineffective solutions. This will be important to take account of in developing workable solutions.

The belief systems and styles of information processing, specified in the second column of the model, which emerge from inquiries about cognitive factors that constrain system members from breaking out of the cycle of interaction around the problem, will suggest fruitful areas for intervention. Alternative belief systems may be co-constructed and new styles of information processing may be developed. In some cases it may be appropriate for some members of a family system to engage in individual therapy to clarify or change their belief systems or styles of information processing.

Predisposing factors in the left hand column of the model provide a way for clinicians to incorporate research on risk factors into their case management plans. This is particularly important in cases of child abuse, marital violence and suicide.

SUMMARY

In Positive Practice the therapist must plan in detail both who to invite to the first session and also what to ask them. The core of the agenda for the intake interview is based on a preliminary formulation of the problem. The three column model is used to develop this preliminary formulation. In the right hand column of this model, the suspected pattern of interaction containing the presenting problem in which the problem-person and members of the problem-system are caught up, is set out. In the left hand column, factors which it is suspected predispose participants in this cycle to persist in this repetitive sequence of interaction are noted. In the central column, suspected beliefs or styles of information processing which mediate the influence of predisposing factors on the present cycle of activity are listed. Lines of inquiry which allow the therapist to test hypotheses entailed by the preliminary formulation are listed and form the core of the agenda for the first session. Other important items on the agenda for the first session are dealing with any possible engagement difficulties and forming a contract for the assessment process. In Positive Practice, the therapist uses the method described in Chapter 2 for mapping out the roles played by members of the problem-system to identify any possible engagement difficulties. The stage-based developmental model of the consultation process, described in Chapter 1, forms a framework for the therapist to plan how to establish and embark upon a contract for assessment with the family in the first session.

Exercise 3.1.

Work in pairs.

Base this exercise on a new referral that has come to you this week or on the Dawn Rooney case first mentioned in Exercise 2.1.

Develop a preliminary three column formulation and an interview plan for the intake interview.

Note those areas in which you are competent and those areas in which you feel challenged.

When you have drawn up your formulation and interview plan, compare it with others in the group.

4

Developing an Assessment Contract

FORMING AN ASSESSMENT CONTRACT WITH THE BARROWS

Mr Dick Barrow, Mrs Sheila Barrow, Caroline, and her only sibling, Mat, attended the intake interview. The main goal of the first section of the interview was to establish a contract for assessment. Subsidiary goals included developing a good working alliance with family members, but with Mr Barrow in particular and defining the neutral role of the clinic with respect to the family and other involved agencies. These objectives were in keeping with the plan outlined in Chapter 3.

I began by shaking hands with Mr Barrow and asking him to introduce me to the other people in the family. I then moved on to explain my understanding of the referral process to him, before addressing the other members of the family. In doing so, I mentioned both referral letters and checked that all four family members knew that Caroline had been simultaneously referred by both the paediatrician and by the educational psychologist. The fact that the school system was construing Caroline's difficulty as misconduct and was threatening to take legal action was contrasted with the paediatrician's view of Caroline as suffering from a psychosomatic problem. I mentioned that our clinic was independent of both the Paediatric and Education departments and would take a neutral stance in relation to the legal issue if we became involved. The involvement of a large number of professionals in the case, and the fact that their involvement had limited impact on Caroline's condition was noted. In light of this I then asked Mr Barrow directly if he wanted yet another agency involved. He said he had not met the other involved professionals but that he wanted the problem sorted out now. I said that that was my impression from the start, because he had taken time off work to come to the clinic with his family. I then asked for his permission to interview the family. He said "Yes. Let's get on with this. That's what we're here for."

Mrs Barrow, Mat and Caroline were asked who they thought was most concerned about the problem. Then each was asked to rank order all family members in terms of

31

their concern about the problem and its resolution. There was a consensus that Mrs Barrow was the most concerned, Caroline, the next most concerned, and the men were joint third with respect to this issue. I then said that there was a high level of concern about the problem among all family members and that this was a good prognostic sign. Each member of the family was then asked if they were willing to participate in a two hour assessment interview. I explained that all family members would be interviewed together and that if individual interviews were necessary they would be conducted at another time. The preliminary assessment interview, it was explained, would lead to a clear plan for completing assessment and planning a strategy for managing the problem. It was also mentioned that assessments rarely exceeded three interviews. All four family members agreed to this.

During this agreement process, I asked explicit permission to use first names. This led to a change in atmosphere from formal and guarded to informal and relatively open.

THE PROBLEM OF PERIPHERAL FATHERS

Structural family therapists, most notably Minuchin, have drawn our attention to a pattern of family organisation where the mother and child have a close alliance to which the father is peripheral (Colapinto, 1991; Minuchin, 1974). This pattern is common where the child is ill or has problems that precipitate a referral for therapy. Fathers who participate in this pattern of family organisation are often referred to as *peripheral fathers*, and it is part of the family therapy lore that these peripheral fathers are particularly difficult to engage in therapy. It is believed that they contribute little to child-focused family interviews and frequently miss appointments.

A wider analysis of the problem of peripheral fathers is important because there is a danger that therapists will blame fathers for being peripheral and for not becoming involved in therapy. This blaming will reinforce their already alienated position. Families that contain peripheral fathers usually live in our Western culture where the sex-role requirements and values lead fathers, for the most part, to work outside the home and mothers to work within the home. Thus, peripheral fathers live in a culture that separates them from their children. Furthermore, it is common practice for most clinics to offer appointments during office hours when peripheral fathers are at work, and not to offer appointments when peripheral fathers are available. Thus, the way we therapists organize service delivery reinforces fathers' alienation from the consultation process.

A key task in family therapy is to engage peripheral fathers. With the Barrows this task was at the top of our agenda. We quite accurately guessed that Mr Barrow was peripheral to previous attempts to resolve Caroline's difficulty. He had not met any of the other involved professionals. Our overriding strategy was to address him *as if* he wanted to be deeply involved in attempting to resolve the problem. In doing so, we would construct together a view of the problem and its solution in which Mr Barrow would play an important part.

This issue of engaging peripheral fathers in therapy is important because a substantial amount of research shows that father-involvement is a major factor in determining the success of family therapy where the child is the presenting problem (Gurman and Kniskern, 1978). Where fathers are engaged in therapy and where they view the therapist as active and competent in directing the therapy process in its early stages, the chances of successful resolution of the presenting problem are increased (Bennun, 1989).

From a feminist perspective, the approach used to engage Mr Barrow may be criticised for reinforcing a patriarchal view of the family's power structure (McGoldrick et al, 1989). This is fair comment. However, it is difficult to engage peripheral fathers without taking this approach. Once the therapist has engaged the father and other family members, more egalitarian approaches to problem-solving may be explored. For example, the task given at the close of the session (and elaborated in Chapter 6) invited Mr and Mrs Barrow to discuss jointly a series of issues on an equal footing.

THE PROBLEM OF NEUTRALITY

Describing the route of referral in detail, the core themes in referral letters, and explicitly outlining the relationship between the clinic, other involved agencies and the family are first steps towards establishing the therapist's neutrality (Selvini-Palazzoli et al, 1980a). If this is not done, problems may occur during contracting because a member of the family may believe that the therapist is not impartial. For example, if Mr Barrow had believed that our function was to provide the Education department with evidence to support a court case against the parents then he might not agreed to an assessment. A number of such engagement difficulties have been outlined in Chapter 2.

THE CUSTOMER QUESTION

In Chapter 2 we identified the customer as a key person in the problem-system. The customer is the one person who most wants the presenting problem to be solved. When a moderately well functioning family are referred for therapy because of child-focused problems, the customer is often the mother. With chaotic and severely dysfunctional families, a social worker is usually the customer. In medical settings, the customer is often the referring physician or surgeon.

However, customerhood is not a stable all-or-nothing state attributable to only one system-member. Everybody in the problem-system at any one time can be placed on a continuum from being a 100% customer to being a 0% customer. deShazer (1988) identifies three important points on this continuum: customers, complainers and visitors. Customers want to change and are receptive to following advice on how to behave productively in problem situations. Complainers are upset by the problem and want to talk about it, but are only receptive to cognitive tasks which require them to develop new ways of thinking about the problem. Visitors are usually sent for consultation (by a parent, spouse or social worker) and have no desire to solve the problem. They are not responsive to any intervention, so deShazer advises simply treating them respectfully in case they should one day evolve into customers.

One way to assess customerhood, illustrated in the interview with the Barrows, is to ask the customer question:

• *Who is most concerned about the problem?*

This is then followed up with questions inquiring about the rank ordering of people within the system in terms of concern. Customerhood can be assessed from time to time over the course of a series of consultation sessions. The way of viewing the world that the therapist and family construct over the course of therapy will help family members to evolve different degrees of customerhood.

CONTRACTING FOR ASSESSMENT

If all family members have some degree of customerhood, the therapist can offer a contract for assessment to each family member. That is, the therapist can reach a verbal agreement with each person that they will participate in the session. This agreement must include a simple explanation of the duration, style and scope of the interview, and what type of follow-up typically occurs.

It is important that the therapist dispel misconceptions and describe in fairly concrete terms what an assessment session is. A common misconception that parents have, is that the therapist will see the child individually for some procedure that will either change the child's behaviour, alleviate the child's symptoms or yield a diagnosis. Such procedures are imagined to include scolding the child, being sympathetic to the child, hypnotising the youngster, giving medication, or conducting a psychometric assessment. Common misconceptions that children have are that the therapist will put them into care, admit them to hospital or conduct a painful medical procedure.

If one or more family members are not customers and have come to the intake session but do not want to be there, it is important not to proceed with the assessment without dealing with the issue. If the non-customer is a parent, it may be useful to meet with the parents only for ten minutes, and to deal with their reservations. Explain what the assessment will involve, how long it will last and what the non-customer might get out of it. If the non-customer is a child, offer the same explanation in the full family session. In either case, suggest that the non-customer simply watch the assessment process rather than participate. Periodically, offer the non-customer a chance to comment on whether they think the assessment that is emerging is fair and accurate. In one case, a teenage boy came to all assessment and therapy sessions but never agreed to a contract to be involved. However, towards the end of every session he offered an opinion about therapeutic progress which was very productive.

FORMALITY AND STYLE

With the Barrows, when contracting was completed, I intentionally adopted a more informal style. I asked permission to use first names and this informality changed the atmosphere of the interview. Within an informal atmosphere, it is usually easier for me to participate in a conversation with greater emotional range. This opens more possibilities for understanding the situation, and for later exploration of new ways of construing and dealing with the problem. This, however, is a personal preference.

Other clinicians may prefer a more formal style. The important issue is to develop a style with which you feel comfortable, and which allows you to complete the tasks of assessment and therapy.

CONTRACTING PROBLEMS

A number of events may complicate the contracting process. The problems of non-attendance and inaccurate referral information are two of the more important obstacles to establishing a contract for assessment with the relevant members of the problem-system.

1. Total non-attendance

When none of the people invited to the intake interview attend, phone the person that you have identified as the customer immediately and clarify why the family have not shown up. Non-attendance, in our experience, may be due either to practical difficulties or to a failure to analyse accurately the roles of members of the problem-system and to identify the customer. Non-attendance due to an inaccurate analysis of the problem system is best dealt with by arranging a meeting with the referrer. This issue has already been discussed in Chapter 2, in the section on engagement mistakes.

Non-attendance due to practical problems occurs most frequently with chaotic families. Chaotic families may lose their appointment letter, be unable to arrange adequate transport or fail to find the clinic. Where practical difficulties lead to non-attendance, families may be offered a home-based intake interview or transport to the clinic. The NHS hospital where some of our work was conducted had a fleet of volunteer drivers and these helped transport some of our clients to intake interviews. When this could not be arranged, assessment sessions were conducted in clients' homes.

2. Partial non-attendance

A second difficulty that complicates the contracting process is when only some of the people invited attend the first session. In statutory cases, where the social worker and the family have been invited to an intake interview, it is not uncommon for the social worker to turn up but for the family to fail to attend. In these cases, a contract for assessment may be formed with the social worker, and the session used to construct a three column formulation insofar as that is possible. The social worker may then be coached on how to help the family engage in the consultation process. Often the simplest option is for the social worker to be coached to explain to the parents of the family the benefits of the consultation process, from the family's viewpoint, and to arrange transportation for the family to come to the next session.

In non-statutory cases, the mother and child often attend the first appointment but the father does not. In such cases, there was a practice at one time for some family therapists to refuse to see families where fathers did not show up (and in line with our earlier discussion of peripheral fathers, to blame all of the family difficulties on the father's peripherality). This strategy is not used in Positive Practice. Rather, the therapist forms a contract to complete an assessment with the mother and child but highlights at the end of the first session the gaps in the formulation that may only be filled by obtaining the father's perspective on the problem. The mother is then coached in how to convey to her husband how his input is vital to the completion of the assessment. If he still does not attend, the therapist may call him directly during the session and offer a contract for assessment on the phone.

Paul Stuart, aged nine, was referred by the GP who identified encopresis (involuntary passing of faeces), attainment problems and disobedience at home as the main problems. He attended the first session with his mother and two older brothers. His father, although invited, did not attend. The mother and the three boys completed an intake interview which led to the construction of an incomplete three column formulation of the problem, presented in Figure 4.1. At the end of the first session I drew this on the whiteboard and highlighted the gaps in the formulation which only Paul's father could complete. I then asked Mrs Stuart to explain to her husband that these gaps in the assessment could only be filled with his help, and therefore that his attendance at the next meeting was important if the consultation process was to proceed and Paul's problems were to be resolved. Mr Stuart did not attend the next session, so I phoned him at the factory where he worked and explained the formulation to him on the phone. I then asked if he would be available later that day, after 5.30 pm, to help complete the picture. He agreed. Mr Stuart attended all subsequent sessions, contributed to the

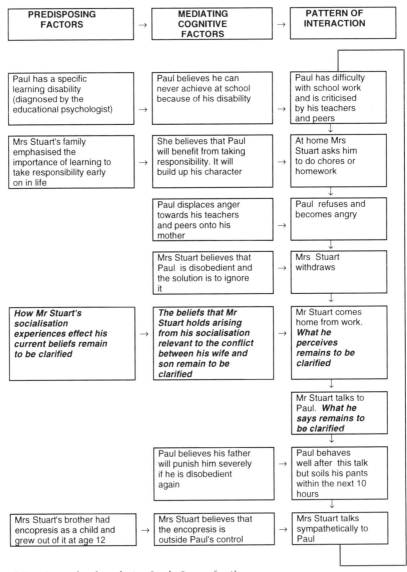

Figure 4.1.   Incomplete formulation for the Stuart family

completion of the formulation and played a major role in helping Paul develop control over his soiling. This proactive approach to engaging non-attending family members in therapy has been used with considerable success in the treatment of drug abusers by Stanton and Todd (1982) and by Szapocznik (1989).

3. Lack of referral information

Sometimes only very limited information about a referred case is available. For example, where a clinic accepts self-referrals or offers a crisis intervention emergency service, the therapist often goes into the intake interview with no background information on the basis of which to construct a preliminary formulation or map of the problem-system. In these situations, the therapist must begin by finding out who the members of the problem-system are, and in particular who the customer is. Once this is established the therapist may ask the customer for an outline of the problem for which consultation is required. At this point it may be useful to take a break, map the system, sketch a preliminary formulation and draw up a plan for the assessment interview. In the light of this, the client may be offered a contract for assessment. You may also specify what other members of the problem-system need to be involved for a thorough assessment to be completed. The following case example illustrates how to manage a situation where no referral information is available.

While conducting a school visit to liaise with Steve Hatter, a teacher, about a youngster on my caseload, Marie Burns interrupted and asked that I meet with her and Jennifer Potter, a fifteen year old who was having a panic attack. I helped Jennifer gain control of her anxiety by using relaxation and breathing exercises and reassurance. I then interviewed Jennifer herself and Marie, her teacher, to clarify the membership of the problem-system. The anxiety appeared to be part of a cycle of interaction that involved Jennifer, her mother and her grandparents with whom she lived. Subsequently a referral meeting was arranged by the teacher where I met the mother, the grandparents and Jennifer and offered a contract for assessment.

4. Inaccurate redflag referral information

Sometimes the information contained in the referral letter, or indeed through a referral phone call, is wildly inaccurate. I am not alluding here to those cases where the referral letter contains factual errors concerning the number of children in the family, or the marital status of the parents. Rather, I am referring to those cases where the referral letter describes the main problem as a manageable focal difficulty, such as enuresis (involuntary passing of urine), and halfway into the intake session the parents mention that one of them has a terminal illness or that they have been planning to separate but have not yet mentioned this to anyone.

In Positive Practice, the therapist is always ready to hear the unexpected and always ready to discard a carefully constructed preliminary formulation and session agenda. When clients indicate that the referral problem was only a red flag to mark a profound life difficulty, the therapist must acknowledge this and acknowledge the validity of the client using a small problem as a way of checking out the therapist's trustworthiness before mentioning the most pressing difficulty. Recontracting for personal or marital work is usually deferred until after the child-focused problems have been dealt with. However, in redflag cases such recontracting may occur in the middle of the first session.

Janice, a widow, and the mother of a girl who had been referred to me previously for neuropsychological testing following a road traffic accident, phoned and requested a referral because her daughter, Eileen, was continuing to have school based difficulties. During the intake interview Janice began to weep uncontrollably and confessed that she had recently been diagnosed as having breast cancer. Dealing with grief associated with this became the core issue for which a therapeutic contract was offered. A routine phonecall to the school, incidentally, revealed that Eileen's progress was adequate, given the constraints placed upon her by the neuropsychological sequelae of the closed head injury she had suffered three years previously.

SUMMARY

At the opening of the first consultation session the therapist describes his understanding of the way the referral occurred and highlights his neutrality with respect to the rest of the problem-system. The therapist then offers a contract for assessment, briefly describing what it will entail and dispelling any misconceptions. Throughout these first few minutes of the session the therapist makes a point of joining with peripheral or alienated members of the problem-system. In non-statutory cases this usually means making a special effort to involve fathers. In statutory cases, both parents may feel more peripheral to the process than the referring social worker. Once the contracting has occurred, some therapists may find it useful to adopt a more informal style. This can make the assessment process less stressful for the family and more fruitful in terms of developing a useful formulation. Partial or total non-attendance and incomplete or inaccurate information are the main problems associated with the contracting phase of consultation. Positive Practice provides the therapist with strategies for dealing with these difficulties.

Exercise 4.1.

Work in groups of at least five members. Four people take the roles of family members described below. The remaining person takes the role of the therapist whose task is to offer an assessment contract to the family on the basis of the information in the referral letter presented below.

People role-playing family members need to take 10 minutes to talk together as a family and develop their roles. The therapist needs to take 10 minutes to plan the way in which he or she will manage the process of offering a contract.

Take about 10 minutes to role-play, offering the therapy contract. Derole after the interview and take 20 minutes to discuss
1.   What the experience was like for family members and
2.   Which aspects of the interviewing process were within the therapist's competence and which offered the greatest challenge.

Referral letter

Dear Therapist

Re: Timmy Whitefriar (Aged 11).

Timmy is one of a pair of fraternal twins. Recently he has been having difficulty sleeping and is not doing well at school. His problems are really not serious but both of his parents are overanxious and want him seen. Please offer them an appointment.

Yours sincerely

Dr Bradley Roundstone
Family Doctor

Family roles

Mother is in her mid-thirties and thinks that Timmy is depressed. She wants some type of solution to this.

Father thinks Timmy is going through a phase and will grow out of it.

Timmy has private reasons for his difficulties which you may make up yourself.

Rex (the other twin) has similar problems to Timmy's which have gone unnoticed.

5

Assessment Part 1
The Cycle of Interaction Around the
Presenting Problem

The objective of the first part of the assessment with the Barrows was to clarify the presenting problem and establish the cycle of interaction that surrounded it. A hypothesis about this cycle of interaction was developed in the right hand column of Figure 3.1. This hypothesis is represented here, for convenience, in Figure 5.1. It was also our intention to identify exceptional circumstances where the problem did not occur.

I began by asking Dick to describe in detail an incident where Caroline developed abdominal pains and was unable to attend school. He said he was unable to do this

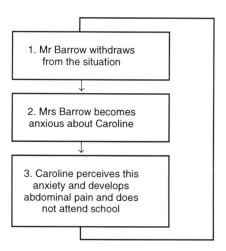

Figure 5.1. Hypothesis about the pattern of interaction around the symptom

41

because he had never observed an incident. He worked as a travelling salesman and usually left home early on Monday and returned late on Friday. (I made a mental note that this was an important issue to come back to after I had clarified the cycle of interaction around the problem.) I then asked Sheila to give a blow by blow account of what usually happened. She gave a vague answer "Caroline sometimes just isn't well. I know she is not. I worry about her. So it's important that she stays in bed". I inquired again and got another vague answer.

So I asked Sheila to select one particular morning in the past ten days and to describe what had happened from the time she got up until about 10 am. Sheila found this easier, and with occasional probing and summarising gave the following picture. Sheila got up first on Thursday. She was worried that Caroline might be unwell again because she did not look well the night before. She went into Caroline's room and asked her if she was all right. Caroline mumbled something and Sheila said "Yes I thought so. I thought you didn't look well last night". Sheila asked Caroline if she wanted breakfast and she said that she did not. Then Sheila said that she had to eat or she would not get better. Caroline whined "I just don't feel like it". Sheila said "Well, see how you feel when you come down". Caroline objected to this and there was a brief argument. Then Sheila went down to make breakfast. Mat was studying in the kitchen, completing a homework assignment and drinking coffee. Sheila made some toast and fried up some bacon and eggs for herself and Mat and Caroline. When Caroline came down Mat and Sheila were eating.

Sheila tried to convince Caroline to eat but she would not. In the end she ate some toast, went up to brush her teeth, had an attack of nausea and vomited. Sheila rushed up to see how Caroline was and insisted that she stay in bed. She lay on her bed in her clothes dozing for an hour and then got up and helped Sheila with the housework.

I then asked Caroline if this fitted in with her recollection of Thursday morning. She said that it did. I asked her what she thought and how she felt

1. when she woke up
2. when Sheila first asked her how she felt
3. at breakfast
4. after breakfast
5. when doing the housework.

She said she had cramps when she woke up. She said they could have been hunger cramps or something else. She said the pain got worse when Sheila asked her about it. It intensified during breakfast but went after she had vomited and did not return for the rest of the day. I integrated this information with Sheila's account and re-presented it to the Barrows. I specifically asked Mat if this fitted in with his observations. Mat agreed that this was what he had seen. I then asked if he ever became involved in the exchanges between Caroline and Sheila. He said that occasionally he would ask Sheila to stop interrogating Caroline about her health and just let her be. Usually this would lead to an argument between Mat and Sheila which would conclude with Sheila shouting and Mat withdrawing. I summarised this cycle of interaction and checked that Sheila, Caroline and Mat believed it to be an accurate account of a typical episode. After they agreed that it represented a typical episode, I put it up on the whiteboard in the office. This is reproduced in Figure 5.2.

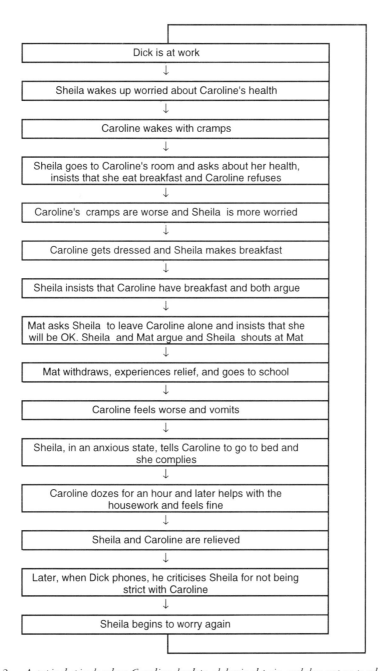

Figure 5.2.   A typical episode where Caroline develops abdominal pain and does not go to school

FOCUSING AN INTERVIEW

In this segment of the intake interview with the Barrows, all of the questions were focused on eliciting information relevant to the cycle of interaction surrounding the presenting problem. Many interesting alternative avenues of inquiry presented them-selves. For example, the circumstances that led Dick to be working in a job that kept him away from home for five days a week and the effects of this on family life generally; or Caroline's medical history; or Mat's career plans. However, a decision was made to focus this section of the interview exclusively on the cycle of interaction around the problem so other leads were mentally noted but not pursued.

In certain situations it is particularly difficult to focus an interview. With large families, holding a focus is difficult because there are many people offering alternative avenues of inquiry. In chaotic families where the parents and children have poor impulse control and freely express a range of intense emotions such as anger, frustration, anxiety and sadness, attempts to help the family focus on a specific issue may intensify their expression of emotion and lead to a further defocusing of the interview.

With both large and chaotic families, it is particularly important to have a clear interview plan. It is difficult to hold a focus, if you are unclear about what that focus should be. Second, before focusing the interview on a specific issue, tell the family your intentions and the rationale for focusing on that issue. For example, with the Barrows I said

- *I'd like to start by finding out about those situations where Caroline gets stomach pains and has difficulty going to school. I need to understand blow-by-blow what happens in a typical situation before I can begin to think about ways of helping you deal with these difficulties.*

Giving the rationale is important because it dispels misconceptions that family members may have about the assessment session. For example, they may think that it is an opportunity for emotional catharsis or a forum for parents to scold children. The importance of giving a rationale for a particular line of interviewing is highlighted by evidence from studies on patients' compliance with medical advice which indicates that patients co-operate with investigations and treatment more readily when they are given the rationale for the procedures (Carr, 1990c).

Third, if a family member wants to discuss a specific issue tangential to the focus of the interview, acknowledge the importance of the issue and put it on the agenda for later in the assessment process. Fourth, if a client has a strong need to express anxiety, sadness, anger, or relief, allow some space for this ventilation and acknowledge that this is what you are doing. For example, in the interview with the Barrows, Sheila became agitated and tearful when she was talking about hearing Caroline vomiting, so I said

- *I know you are really worried about her. Take some time to talk about that if you need to. We can get back on track in a few minutes.*

Finally, it is important to accept that sometimes it is not possible to focus a family interview. In these situations, acknowledge that and suggest that individuals or subgroups be interviewed separately. For example, in a family with seven children, the parents were demanding that one of the children be taken into care. The father's aggression in the family interview made it difficult to focus, so he and his wife were offered separate individual interviews. The children were interviewed as two subgroups. Then, a family meeting was convened where a tentative formulation based on what was said in these four separate meetings was given. The tentative formulation was further refined during this whole-family-meeting and a contract for further consultation offered based on this formulation.

CONSTRUCTING AN INTERACTIONAL DESCRIPTION OF THE PROBLEM

The process of clarifying the presenting problem and then inquiring about the typical sequence of behaviour in which it is embedded, helps the family move from an individual to an interactional way of construing their difficulties.

Certain interviewing tactics are particularly useful in developing an interactional construction of the problem. The first is to follow-up vague answers with probes about specific details. For example, when Sheila gave a vague answer about Caroline's stomach pains, I asked her to select a specific episode that she could remember and then encouraged her to describe this in detail. Throughout her description I summarised the blow-by-blow sequence of events periodically and asked

• *What happened next?*

This approach to interviewing often referred to as "tracking", was pioneered by Minuchin (1974) in the family therapy field, and holds a good deal in common with behavioural approaches to family interviewing (Herbert, 1987).

The second interviewing tactic is to summarise one family member's description of the pattern of interaction in which the presenting problem is embedded and then ask each family member to modify or expand it. Where disagreements occur about the sequence of interaction, a useful tactic is to ask a relatively uninvolved member of the family to comment on the interaction they observe between two or three key members. So, for example, Mat was asked on a number of occasions to clarify details of the pattern of interaction that occurred between Sheila and Caroline. This style of interviewing was popularised in the family therapy field by the original Milan team (Selvini-Palazzoli et al, 1980a) although it has always been widely used by therapists working within a behavioural framework (Herbert, 1987).

Finally, it is useful to offer the family a visual representation of the pattern of interaction around the problem as an aide-mémoire. The visual map of the pattern of interaction on a whiteboard or flipchart can serve as a reference point for other aspects of the assessment. So, for example, we shall see how inquiries about Dick's absence from the family or Sheila's anxiety were directly related to the map of the pattern of interaction around the problem presented in Figure 5.2.

BEHAVIOUR, FEELINGS AND BELIEFS

The pattern or interaction around the presenting problem should only contain statements about how family members *behave* and how they *feel*. The beliefs and intentions that underpin these actions and feelings are placed in the middle column of the three column model.

This segregation of behaviour and feelings on the one hand from belief on the other is, of course, quite artificial. However, there are a number of reasons why doing this and then focusing on the pattern of interaction around the problem in the first part of the assessment is particularly useful. Here are some of the reasons for this approach.

First, family members usually find it relatively easy to describe the sequence of behaviour around the problem and relatively difficult to articulate their belief systems. Interviewing about the pattern of interaction around the problem as the first step in the assessment, therefore, gives family members a sense of mastery within the context of the assessment process from the outset. Second, family members typically find it easy to agree about behavioural patterns that they observe or to accept private emotions and feelings that other members claim to experience. Disagreements are usually about the way in which situations are construed, beliefs that different members hold and the morality of their intentions. By focusing on behaviours and feelings in the early stages of assessment and postponing the exploration of the contentious area of beliefs and intentions, the therapist is helping to create a co-operative climate. Third, in Positive Practice goals are usually stated in terms of changes in behaviour or feelings. So the pattern of interaction around the problem provides a focus for developing goals. Goal setting will be discussed in more detail in Chapter 8.

INTERVIEWING ABOUT EXCEPTIONS

Once the map outlined in Figure 5.2 was in place, I suggested that we construct a list of exceptional situations where the problem does not occur. I began by asking each family member to recall a specific morning where Caroline was not ill and went to school. Dick recalled a Monday morning about six weeks previously where he was attending a meeting at head office in town and so did not have to leave until 9.30 a.m. On that day he had breakfast with the family and Caroline was fine.

Mat mentioned a series of occasions where Kirsty called for Caroline at 8.30 a.m, and she and Caroline went to school together without any problem. Caroline said that some mornings she felt just fine and did not argue with Sheila about having breakfast. I asked Sheila, Dick and Mat if they could offer any explanation for this spontaneous feeling of well-being that Caroline talked about. They gave vague answers like "It could just be the weather. You know some days you wake up and the sun is out and you feel good". I probed for specific factors that might account for Caroline's good mornings to no avail. I then asked Sheila if there were mornings when she awoke and found she was not worrying about Caroline. She said there were but could not pinpoint anything that distinguished these from mornings where she did worry. When the other three family members were asked for their hunches about why some mornings Sheila did not worry about Caroline, Mat had an important observation. He said that when Mary, her closest friend, had visited the day before or was going to visit that day Sheila did not worry about Caroline.

I then checked in summary if it was the case that Caroline did not experience pain and miss school on those occasions when Dick was present, when Sheila had or was going to see Mary and when Tracy called for Caroline. The Barrows agreed that these were the exceptional circumstances where the problem did not occur.

In response to a series of questions about a typical day at school and a typical weekend day, Caroline confirmed that she never experienced abdominal pains while in school or at the weekend. She had been examined by the school nurse (Nurse Boyd) and by the school doctor (Dr Reed) when she was asymptomatic at the request of a teacher who was concerned about her absences and related illness. As has already been mentioned, in the educational psychologist's referral letter, they gave her a clean bill of health.

EXCEPTIONS AND SOLUTIONS

Exceptions are particularly important because they may contain the seeds of a solution. Both behaviour therapists and solution focused therapists emphasise the importance of exploring exceptions (e.g. de Shazer, 1985, 1988; White and Epston, 1990; Herbert, 1987). Behaviour therapists may identify stimuli which elicit problem behaviour and distinguish these from relatively similar stimuli which do not elicit problem behaviour. These stimuli may be identified by asking family members in detail about the antecedents of problem behaviours or by directly observing the family in situations that do and do not elicit the presenting problem. Behavioural treatment programmes based on stimulus control involve replacing stimuli that elicit problem behaviour with stimuli that do not. For example, a young, electively mute girl could speak in the presence of her mother but not at school in the presence of her peers and teacher. A series of situations intermediate between being alone with her mother and being in the class with her peers and teacher were arranged, and in these exceptional circumstances the girl began to speak (Carr and Afnan, 1989). Behavioural treatments such as systematic desensitisation involve training children to overcome their anxiety through the use of relaxation training by moving gradually from situations which do not elicit anxiety to those that do.

deShazer, a pioneering solution-focused therapist bases his approach to therapy on amplifying exceptional sequences of interaction where the problem does not occur (deShazer, 1985, 1988). He asks clients first to identify pretreatment changes. These are changes that clients experience in the frequency or intensity of the problem between requesting a referral and attending the first session. He then inquires about the circumstances surrounding them, and whether the changes were experienced by the clients as within or outside their control. In the light of this information he invites clients between sessions to investigate further the conditions under which exceptions occur, or to carry out tasks that make it likely that exceptions will recur. For example, a boy who often got into trouble with his mother after access visits with his father, noted that this sometimes did not occur. When asked about the circumstances under which these exceptions occurred, the boy and his mother guessed that it was when his father drove him home, and told his mother what he had done during the visit although he was not sure. The boy and his mother were asked to try to predict if they would fight after the next two access visits.

White (1993) invites clients to externalise their problems rather than identify with them. For example, he asked a single-parent who was having difficulties with her daughter, to take the idea " a failure as a mother" and explore how she had been recruited into accepting this external definition as a central part of her identity. He then helped her to identify what he refers to as *unique outcomes*. These are situations where she resisted accepting a definition of herself as a failed mother. He invited her then to historicize these unique outcomes by tracing back through her own development situations where she had refused to accept a self definition of being a failure.

All three of these approaches involve identifying situations where the cycle of interaction around the presenting problem could have happened but did not because of exceptional circumstances. In all three approaches, the identification of the exception contains the seeds of a solution. The use of exceptions as a basis for developing homework tasks to break the cycle of interaction around the presenting problem, or as a way of helping clients manage resistance to change, will be discussed in Chapters 9 and 10.

MULTIPROBLEM FAMILIES

Multiproblem families deserve special mention. In public hospital clinics and public social service agencies, they form a numerically significant part of most therapists' caseloads and consume a major portion of therapists time and energy (e.g. Carr, McDonnell and Owen, 1994).

Often the fact that families have multiple problems does not emerge until the therapist tries to track the pattern of interaction around the presenting problem. Maintaining focus then becomes extremely difficult because one problem is piled on top of the next until therapist and family feel overwhelmed by the number and the complexity of the problems. Attempting to accommodate all of such a family's problems within a simple three column formulation, while possible, is probably not useful.

In Positive Practice, the therapist and the family acknowledge this, and avoid becoming overwhelmed by eating the proverbial elephant in thin slices. First, all of the family problems are listed. They are then clumped into meaningful bunches of difficulties. These clumps are then prioritised. Once this has been done, the therapist offers a contract for consultation focusing on the first clump only, leaving open the possibility of recontracting.

For example, the Floods were referred because eight year old Colin stole thirty pounds from his mother. While the pattern of interaction around the problem was being clarified, other problems were mentioned. These were listed and clumped into the following bunches:

Clump 1. Colin and Mark's stealing, lying and disobedience
Clump 2. Sarah's bedwetting
Clump 3. Mrs Flood's low mood and lack of social support
Clump 4. Mr Flood's erratic approach to access visits with the boys

Mrs Flood was adamant that the first clump was her major concern and the first contract for consultation focused on these difficulties. Of course, some of the problems in clumps 2, 3, and 4 were included in the formulation of the clump 1 problems, but the central focus was Colin and Mark's antisocial behaviour. The formulation for the first episode of consultation with the Flood family is presented in Figure 5.3.

SUMMARY

Once the family have accepted a contract for assessment, the first part of the assessment involves the therapist clarifying, in specific terms, the presenting problem and the cycle

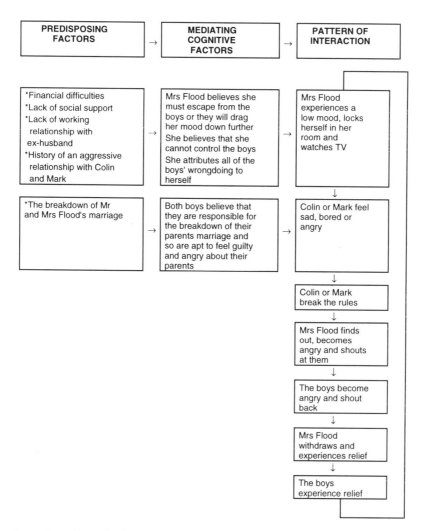

Figure 5.3. Formulation for the first clump of problems in the Flood family

of interaction that surrounds it. A style of questioning that specifically inquires into what happens before, during, and after the occurrence of the problem during a typical episode is used in Positive Practice. Where major discrepancies between accounts of the problem are given by different family members, relatively uninvolved members of the family may be asked to comment on what they observe other family members to be doing during a problem episode. The goal is to construct a consensualy agreed description of the typical cycle of interaction which surrounds the presenting problem when it occurs, which may be placed in the right hand column of the three column formulation model. The pattern surrounding the presenting problem contains descriptions of behaviour or experienced emotions. Accounts of family members' beliefs are not included in this column of the formulation. They are placed in the middle column of the model.

A major challenge during the assessment process is to maintain focus and to avoid straying from the pursuit of this goal. Vague answers or a reluctance to speak on the one hand, or highly detailed simultaneous contributions from many family members on the other are among the more common factors that deflect therapists from maintaining focus. Keeping the goal of this section of the assessment in mind, and using a style of interviewing which is directed towards this goal are central to maintaining focus. It is also important to give family members your rationale for doing so. A further factor which challenges the therapists attempt to maintain focus is extreme emotional reactions.

It is not uncommon for family members to experience extreme emotional reactions of anger, sadness or fear during the assessment process. In Positive Practice, clients are given space to ventilate these feelings before guiding the interview back to the central focus of establishing the cycle of interaction around the problem.

Once this has been constructed, exceptional episodes where one would expect the problem to occur but it does not, are identified and factors that typify these exceptional episodes are brought to light.

If multiple problems emerge during this part of the assessment process, these may be listed, clumped, and the clumps of problems prioritised. Then, one clump is assessed at a time. This, process prevents the therapist and the family from becoming overwhelmed by the number and complexity of the presenting difficulties.

Exercise 5.1.

This exercise is based on the Whitefriar case described in Exercise 4.1.

Work in groups of at least five members. Four people take the roles of family members. The remaining person or people take the roles of the therapist and team.

The therapist (with preconsultation suggestions from the team) must clarify

1.   The pattern of interaction around the presenting problem
2.   The exceptional patterns of interaction where the problem would be expected to occur but does not.

People role-playing family members need to take 10 minutes to talk together as a family and develop their roles. Therapist and team need to take 10 minutes to plan the way in which the interview will be managed.

Take about 30 minutes to role play the interview.

Derole after the interview.

Take 20 minutes to discuss

1.   What the experience was like for family members and
2.   Problems that were encountered by the therapist in trying to keep the interview focused and what particularly did the therapist do to maintain focus.

6

Assessment Part 2
History and Genogram Construction

Once a detailed interactional description of an episode of the presenting problem has been constructed in the right hand column of the three column formulation model, the next sets of objectives of the assessment process are twofold. First, factors that predispose system members to continue to participate in these episodes in stereotyped ways must be identified. Second, the beliefs and habitual styles of information processing that link these predisposing factors to current behaviour during an episode of problem behaviour must be clarified.

Let us return to the example of the Barrow family. Here, the objectives at this point were to find out answers to these specific questions.

- *Why does Dick believe that he must be absent from the family consistently throughout the week, and what predisposes him to hold this set of beliefs?*
- *What set of beliefs underpin Sheila's deep concern for Caroline's well-being and what events predisposed her to developing these?*
- *What factors predispose Caroline to experiencing nausea, frequent abdominal pain and vomiting; and what beliefs lead her into frequent arguments with Sheila about how best to deal with these symptoms?*
- *What beliefs lead Mat to try unsuccessfully to intervene between Sheila and Caroline periodically, and what types of experiences predispose him to behaving in this way?*

For each of the involved family members, we also wanted to determine if particular styles of information processing or defences were being used to strengthen or potentiate the beliefs that underpinned family members' roles in the pattern of interaction surrounding the presenting problem. We also wished to identify the events that predisposed family members to using these styles of information processing or defences. Here are some examples of such questions that guided the next step in the assessment of the Barrow family.

51

- *Is Dick using denial or rationalisation to allow him to be absent from family life and if so what predisposes him to do so?*
- *Is Sheila maximising negative features of Caroline's health and minimising positive features, and if so what predisposes her to do so?*

For all of these types of questions, direct lines of inquiry and careful observation of how family members talk about the presenting problem and immediately-related beliefs are important. However, such a direct approach alone may provide too little information to construct a useful formulation of the presenting problem. The therapist may find that he attends to only those aspects of the problem upon which the family are focusing. Direct inquiry may lead the therapist into the same dead-end in which the family is already stuck. Direct inquiry needs to be supplemented with broader assessment methods that address the child's development, the social context of the family and the development of the family over the lifecycle.

Information from this broader inquiry may throw light on predisposing factors, beliefs, information processing styles and defences that would not emerge from direct inquiries alone. In Positive Practice, constructing a developmental history, a family history and a genogram are the three principal methods for broadening the scope of the enquiry.

CONSTRUCTING A DEVELOPMENTAL HISTORY

Four key areas may fruitfully be addressed when constructing a developmental history: first, the pregnancy, second, progression through stages identified by major theories of child development; third, temperament; and fourth, attachment. The order in which these areas are explored will vary from case to case and different therapists will have different preferences. My own preference is to start with the present and work backwards. Family members, in my experience, often find it easier to see the relevance of history taking if the line of inquiry moves gradually from the management of recent difficulties and challenges to the management of earlier developmental tasks. However, it is probably conceptually more coherent to present the frameworks for history construction here beginning with the earliest period of life.

1. Pregnancy

When exploring the events surrounding conception and pregnancy one of the most important concerns is the degree to which the parents wanted a child. Children who are not wanted or whose parents have been desperate to have a child are both at risk for developing adjustment problems. A second issue is whether the pregnancy was easy or difficult and the way this was construed. Where women experience a difficult pregnancy some construe the process as a basis for valuing their child. For example, one mother said "I went through so much for her during the pregnancy, that I feel closer to her than any of the others". In other cases a difficult pregnancy may lead to the mother construing the child negatively. This is typified by the remarks of a second-time mother who said "I've never really felt right about him. It started during that awful time in the first trimester. I felt terrible and was edgy. I felt like he was putting a rift between Anna (the first child) and me". A third concern is the degree to which physical prenatal and perinatal factors place a child at risk for developing difficulties and these should also be explored. Some of the more important factors to take account of are contained in Figure 6.1. A fuller description of these is given in Barker's (1988) excellent child-psychiatry text. (This text is particularly useful for family therapists because Philip Barker, an eminent Child Psychiatrist is also an established family therapist who has practiced on both sides of the Atlantic, e.g. Barker, 1986).

RISK FACTOR	
Maternal age	Below 20 and above 35, risks of congenital defects and birth complications are increased
Blood-type incompatibility	Erethroblastosis due to blood type incompatibility can lead to sensory and cognitive impairment, even if a blood transfusion is given at birth
Prenatal maternal malnutrition	This impairs cognitive development but can be addressed through early stimulation programmes
Maternal drug abuse during pregnancy	Children of drug dependent mothers suffer on two counts. At a physiological level they suffer abstinence symptoms. At a social level their mothers are less responsive than normal mothers. They often show developmental delays in reaching milestones
HIV infected children	These show a variety of neurodevelopmental disorders and slow cognitive and motor development
Perinatal complications	Perinatal brain insult due to forceps delivery can lead to later cognitive impairment. Anoxia at birth (blue babies with low apgars) may suffer brain damage and show later cognitive impairment
Low birthweight	(VLBW1000-1499g; ELBW: 500-999g). These children show later deficits in cognitive, motor and social development. Some are directly attributable to physiological factors and some to parent-child interaction, since LBW children come from disadvantaged families. Dietary treatments and family intervention are indicated here

Figure 6.1.   Prenatal and perinatal risk factors

2. Stages of development

A developmental history gives an account constructed by the therapist and the family of the way in which the child has managed the various physical, cognitive, emotional and interpersonal tasks of development. From the clinician's viewpoint, the child's management of developmental tasks is interpreted in the light of theoretical and empirical literature on normative child development. Thus, the developmental history allows the clinician to judge if the child's development has been, broadly speaking, within normal limits for our culture. Attainment of developmental milestones on time is a protective factor. Children who reach milestones on time are better equipped with the skills they need to manage normal challenges and abnormal stress than those that do not. Children who reach their milestones late are at risk for developing further difficulties because they are ill equipped to manage the challenges and stresses that face them. A summary of the main milestones entailed by major theories of psychological development are set out in Figure 6.2. Mussen's introductory text gives a good summary of the child development literature (Mussen et al, 1990).

STAGE	MAIN ACCOMPLISHMENTS
First year	**Piaget's Sensory-Motor Period** Walking Object constancy Perception of cause and effect **Erikson's Trust V Mistrust Period** Social smile at 3 months Making strange at 8 months Secure attachment by end of first year **Freud's Oral Stage** Routines for eating and sleeping develop
Second year	**Piaget's Sensory Motor Period Continues** Talking in sentences Egocentric view of the world **Erikson's Period of Autonomy Vs Shame and Doubt** Exploration develops and resistance to limits occurs Achievement of some autonomy from parents occurs **Freud's Anal Stage** Bowel and bladder control begins to develop
Pre-school years 2-5 years	**Piaget's Preoperational Period** Language development accelerates Children hold animistic beliefs Fantasy play develops **Erickson's Initiative Vs Guilt Period** The task is to emerge feeling confident about initiating with peers and adults Children learn to separate from attachment figures and attend play-school Transitional objects (Winnicott,1965) are used to deal with separation anxiety **Freud's Genital Stage** The tasks are to develop a sex role, a conscience and a set of defences against anxiety Masturbation and sexplay with siblings and friends occurs Internalisation of parental standards is impaired in some children because of unstable or chaotic relationship with parental figures Repression, rationalisation reaction formation etc. develop to protect the child's ego from anxiety caused by real or imagined threats to himself or his attachment figures
Middle childhood 6-12 years	**Piaget's Concrete Operations Period (7-12)** Learns to internalise properties of objects and mentally sequence or classify them Capacity for empathy (non-egocentric) thinking emerges **Erikson's Industry vs Inferiority Stage** Self-esteem through skill-mastery occurs High self-esteem develops if children master skills at school (reading, writing maths etc.), in the family (doing chores) or in clubs (sports, games or complex hobbies) Low self-esteem develops if skill-mastery fails to occur **Freud's Latency Period** Contrary to Freud's theory, this is not a period of sexual inactivity Masturbation and heterosexual play are common
Adolescence 12-19 years	**Piaget's Formal Operations Period** The ability to construct and test hypotheses develops The ability to identify logical patterns and inconsistencies develops Arguments about adult hypocrisy and careful logical justification for the adolescent's own behaviour occurs **Erikson's Identity vs Role Confusion Stage** Identity formation occurs The adolescent develops * emotional independence from the parents and establishes an adult-adult relationship with them * the capacity to make and maintain lasting peer friendships * a career plan and moving towards economic independence * a personal moral system **Freud's Genital Stage** The development of the capacity for a lasting heterosexual partnership was Freud's primary task here To this may be added the alternative of being able to develop a lasting ego-syntonic homosexual partnership

Figure 6.2.   Child's development history

3. Temperament

The child's temperament, and the extent to which the child's temperamental characteristics fit with the parental expectations, have been found to have far-reaching effects on children's later adjustment. Temperament refers to those characteristic styles of responding with which a child is endowed at birth. Chess and Thomas (1984) identified three distinct and relatively common temperamental profiles and these are described in Figure 6.3. Easy temperament children have a good prognosis. They attract adults and peers to form a supportive network around them. Easy temperament is a protective factor. Difficult temperament children are at risk for developing psychological problems. They have more conflict with parents, peers and teachers. They do better when there is a *goodness-of-fit* between their temperament and the parental expectations. Difficult temperament children need tolerant, responsive parents. Children who are slow-to-warm-up also require more tolerant parents than do easy temperament children, and their prognosis is more variable than the other two temperamental types.

TEMPERAMENTAL TYPE	CHILD'S RESPONSE PATTERN
Easy temperament	Regular in eating, sleeping and eliminating habits Approaches new situations rather than avoids them Adapts to new situations easily Moods are predominantly positive and of low intensity
Difficult temperament	Irregular in eating, sleeping and eliminating habits Avoids new situations Slow to adapt to new situations Moods are predominantly negative and of high intensity
Slow to warm up	Moderately irregular in eating, sleeping and eliminating habits Slow to adapt to new situations Moods are predominantly negative but of low intensity

Figure 6.3.   Temperament

4. Attachment

Ainsworth et al (1978) have distinguished between three different patterns of attachment. These are described in Figure 6.4. Secure attachment to a parent figure is a protective factor. It provides the child with an immediate source of security and a model for developing later supportive relationships. Anxiously attached or anxiously avoidant children are at risk for developing psychological difficulties. They lack an immediate secure base from which to explore their environment. They also lack a model on which to base later socially supportive relationships.

Attachment behaviour and temperament may be directly observed in young children, whereas with older clients, clinicians have to base their assessment of these important constructs on the parents' account of the child's early behaviour.

In our interview with the Barrow family, Sheila described her pregnancy with Caroline as normal. No significant prenatal or perinatal factors were noted. As a young

ATTACHMENT PATTERN	CHILD AND MOTHER'S BEHAVIOUR
Secure attachment	These children seek proximity following separation and explore actively in their mother presence. Their mothers are highly responsive to the child's cues
Anxious attachment	These infants alternate between seeking and avoiding proximity . They can't derive comfort from contact with their mothers. These mothers tend to be unresponsive to children's cues
Anxious-avoidant attachment	These infants resist proximity after separation and do not seek their mothers under stress. They do not seem disturbed when separated. They have usually been treated harshly or rejected so they learn to avoid their mothers but can respond to other adults

Figure 6.4.   Attachment patterns

child she had a slow-to-warm up temperament. She adapted slowly to new situations, but reacted with mild rather than intense emotion. For example, if a neighbour visited, Caroline would be withdrawn and glum looking during her second year of life. She might cry briefly, if asked insistently to approach the neighbour. She formed a good secure attachment to Sheila by the end of her first year. In fact, they were inseparable. Her milestones including walking, talking, toilet training, forming friendships in playschool and the first year of junior school and these were all within normal limits. The only noteworthy feature of middle childhood was her repeated attacks of gastroenteritis, usually in the winter months. She was involved in the brownies and did some horse riding regularly during her period in junior school. Her transition to secondary school was uneventful. Her abdominal pains were unrelated to menstruation which had begun at the age of twelve.

QUESTIONS TO ASK IN CONSTRUCTING A DEVELOPMENTAL HISTORY

In constructing a developmental history, it is useful to divide the child's lifespan into chunks and then to ask about how the tasks in each of these chunks were managed. What follows are clusters of questions appropriate to each of the main developmental stages contained in Figure 6.2, along with questions specifically targeting the areas of attachment and temperament. The groups of questions are not intended as a comprehensive interview schedule, but rather are illustrative of the style of inquiry used for developmental history construction in Positive Practice.

Let us begin with some typical broad questions about the tasks of adolescence.

- *At the moment and up until you are (or your child is) about twenty the main job is developing a sense of independence. How do you see yourself (your child) going about that?*
- *How would you know (your parents know) if you (your child) wanted privacy?*

- *How would you (your child) go about saving up for something you (your child) wanted? Where would the cash come from?*
- *Do you (does your child) have a set of jobs that you (your child) have to do around the house/ a part time job outside the house etc.?*
- *What friends would you (your child) see most often during the week or at the weekend?*
- *Who do you talk to about what you will do when you leave school?*
- *What do you think your parents would like you to do when you graduate and how does that differ from your own plan?*
- *What do you think your child would like to do when he leaves school and how does that differ from your plans?*

The following questions focus on the middle childhood period.

- *You remember primary school. What stands out in your mind about how you (your child) got on then?*
- *How did you (your child) go about making friends at primary school?*
- *What do you remember about your (your child's) school reports in primary school?*

These questions target the preschool period.

- *What are your most vivid memories of your child as a toddler? That is, during the two to five year old period?*
- *How did your child manage at pre-school?*
- *What kinds of friendships did your child have when she was a toddler?*
- *How did your child learn about the difference between right and wrong?*

These questions are useful ways of asking about attachment during the preschool years.

- *How did your child settle when you took him or her to pre-school and then had to leave him or her with the teacher?*
- *When you went visiting, did your child spend most of the time on your knee or would your child go off and explore?*
- *How did your child treat you when you left him or her with a baby-sitter or your mother for a while and then came back?*
- *How long did it take your child to give up using a security blanket or comforter (transitional object)?*

The following questions are useful for asking about the first two years.

- *Let's talk about early milestones. Can you remember if your child sat up, walked and talked, and so on, at the times you would have expected these things to happen?*
- *Did your child's language develop the way you expected it to?*
- *How did your child take to toilet training?*

Here are some questions that relate to the first two years but specifically inquire about temperamental characteristics.

- *How regular was your child in following routines for feeding, sleeping and toileting?*

- *Some children are curious and approach new situations. Others are more cautious and avoid situations that they know nothing about. How was your child when faced with a new situation, like going on a visit to someone else's house?*
- *When your child was doing one thing like playing in the kitchen, and you had to interrupt him or her so that you could go out shopping or move to another room, how would your child react?*

CONSTRUCTING A GENOGRAM

The genogram is a family tree that contains at least three clinically useful types of information. First, it contains information about the membership of the family and related social network. Second, it throws light on sources of social support and stress within the family system. Finally, it points to productive and destructive patterns of relationships within the nuclear and extended family. Not only do genograms provide useful information, but the process of constructing a genogram in a participative manner with a family is a structured way of strengthening the therapeutic alliance.

The process is introduced as a way of providing a broad understanding of how the family copes with ordinary problems of family life, and therefore may throw some light ways of tackling the presenting problem. Using a large sheet of paper or a whiteboard is important, since it allows all family members to have a clear view of the genogram as it develops.

My own preference is to use genograms to engage family members who have found it difficult to become involved in the earlier part of the interview. For example, children and teenagers who have had little say in the early part of the interview may be given the task of drawing the genogram after the rules for using the symbols have been explained to them. With Caroline and Mat, I explained that squares stand for males and circles for females. The names and ages go inside these symbols. Horizontal lines stand for marriage and vertical lines for parent-child relationships. I then sketched the nuclear family on the board (Figure 6.5) and asked them to extend the genogram upwards by filling in the grandparents, and outwards by filling in their aunts and uncles. Where they were unsure about details I encouraged them to ask their parents.

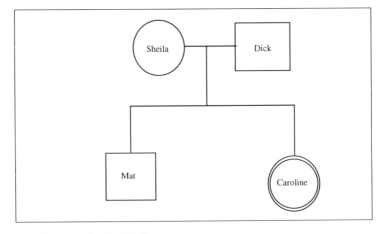

Figure 6.5.   Preliminary sketch of the Barrow's genogram

From time to time they needed more rules to help them code information on the genogram. (All of the genogram rules are contained in Figures 6.6a and 6.6b) For example, June, the maternal grandmother had died in the past eighteen months, so they needed to put an X in her symbol. Also, I asked if there had been other deaths or stillbirths and Sheila mentioned that before Caroline's conception she had had a miscarriage. The appropriate symbol for this was used in the genogram.

There was a digression here, where Sheila was given space to talk about this and be supported. There was also a discussion about how the family coped with this. Sheila said she put it behind her, did not talk about it, and rejoiced when Caroline was born, fit and healthy, a year later. However, she became particularly careful about caring for Caroline's health and well-being as a result of the stillbirth.

I made a mental note here to include the stillbirth in our formulation as a factor that may have predisposed Sheila to hold strong beliefs about Caroline's possible vulnerability to illness. This may have been linked to her treatment of Caroline's presenting problem.

Once the genogram contained all important family members along with their names, ages and occupations, I invited Caroline and Mat to include other important details following the checklist in Figure 6.7. In noting major transitions they recorded that their paternal grandfather had deserted their grandmother when Dick was three years old. Dick had, played a major role in bringing up his two younger brothers. Sheila and Dick had married when they were twenty-nine and thirty-five respectively. Sheila's mother had died in September 1988. No other noteworthy transitions were mentioned.

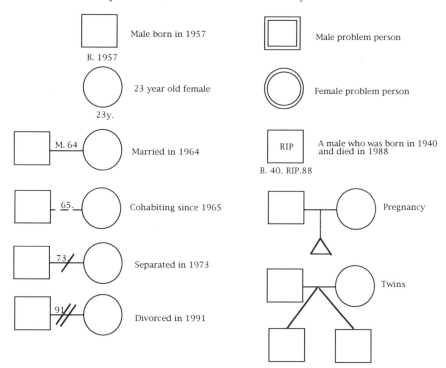

Figure 6.6a.   Genogram symbols

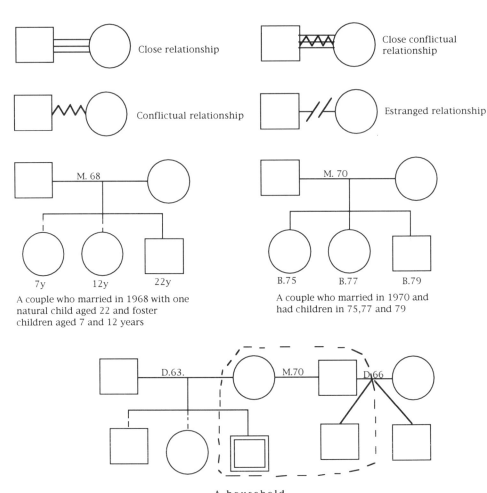

Figure 6.6b.   More genogram symbols

Inquiries about illnesses and psychosocial problems revealed that Sheila's mother had suffered recurrent episodes of depression and had died of cancer.

A number of additional network members were identified who were particularly important. Caroline had a close friend Kirsty who had daily contact with her. On days when Kirsty called for her in the morning she usually went to school without difficulty, even if she awoke with abdominal pains. Sheila had daily contact with Mary, a neighbour, and valued that relationship highly. She also visited the family physician, Dr Wilson, frequently.

The Barrow's nuclear family had limited contact with members of the extended family. They visited the maternal grandfather, Tom, at Christmas and Easter. They saw the paternal grandmother, Annie, about every four months. Sheila and Dick's siblings visited occasionally but neither they, nor their children, were major sources of social support or stress for the Barrow's nuclear family.

An exploration of relationships within the family revealed two interesting patterns. First, within the nuclear family there was a clear triangle with a close cross-generational alliance between Caroline and Sheila, and a weaker and sometimes conflictual relationship between Dick and Sheila. Second, there was a four generational pattern of close mother-daughter relationships. The intense relationship which Caroline and Sheila had was similar to that which Sheila and her mother June had, and that which June had with her mother, May. The Barrow's final genogram is presented in Figure 6.8.

A complete exploration of the use of the genogram in family assessment is given in McGoldrick and Gerson's (1985) text. Numerous interesting examples, including the genograms of Sigmund Freud, Carl Jung and Gregory Bateson are included in this entertaining book.

GENOGRAMS

THE PEOPLE

1. **IDENTIFYING INFORMATION.** Names, ages, dates of birth and occupations

2. **MAJOR TRANSITIONS (ENTRANCES AND EXITS).** Dates of leaving home, moving house, dates of marriage and separation, dates of deaths, adoptions, fostering, stillbirths and anniversary reactions

3. **MAJOR ILLNESSES AND PSYCHOSOCIAL PROBLEMS.** Hospitalisations, serious physical illnesses, psychological problems (such as depression, child abuse, and addiction) and criminality

4. **PROTECTIVE FACTORS.** Personal achievements, skills or ways of coping that may be useful in finding a solution to the problem

THE PATTERNS

4. **OTHER SIGNIFICANT NETWORK MEMBERS.** Close friends, confidants and involved professionals

5. **QUALITY AND QUANTITY OF CONTACT WITHIN THE NETWORK.** Distance between nuclear family and other members of the family and network, frequency of contact and estimation of how supportive or stressful this is

6. **FAMILY FACTIONS AND PATTERNS.** Especially close, conflictual, dependent and estranged relationships; triangles (e.g. mother and child vs father); and multigenerational patterns (e.g. youngest sons include mothers in their family's household for 3 generations)

Figure 6.7.   Information to include in genograms

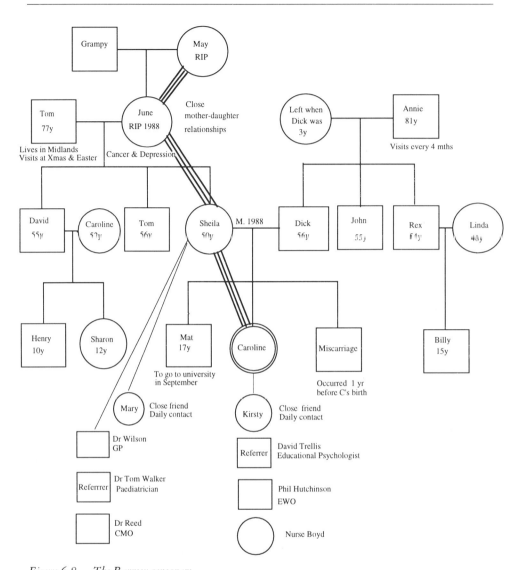

Figure 6.8.   The Barrow genogram

QUESTIONS TO ASK WHEN CONSTRUCTING A GENOGRAM

When constructing a genogram, there are two common pitfalls. The first is to ask too many questions about trivial details. The second is not to ask enough questions about significant patterns.

If family members can not remember ages, dates and occupations, unless you have reason to believe these omissions have a particular significance that is relevant to the presenting problem and their way of coping with it, ignore the omissions.

When asking about illnesses and psychosocial difficulties, ask the question about each generation or the family as a whole, rather than each individual. For example, with the Barrows I asked

- *Has anyone in this generation had a serious illness or been hospitalised (pointing to the grandparents' generation)?*

This was followed with a similar question about the parent's generation and the children's generation. Then, I asked in a colloquial way about psychosocial problems in each generation:

- *Do you know if anyone in this generation had bad nerves or a problem with drink?*

Similar questions were asked of each generation. When inquiring about criminality, because it seemed unlikely to me that anyone in the family had been convicted or imprisoned, I asked the question with reference to the whole family rather than to a single generation

- *Has anyone in the family been in serious trouble with the police?*

To identify other significant members of the network, some useful questions are

- *Outside of the family are there any close friends (neighbours/doctors/teachers etc.) that are important because they are very helpful to you and so should be on the family map?*
- *Are there any people that are important because they cause your family a lot of hassle and so should be on the map?*

To explore the quantity and quality of relationships within the network some questions are useful in keeping this process brief.

- *Which people in the network do you see on a daily basis and which do you see infrequently, like just at Christmas and Easter?*
- *Are these contacts a hassle or are they something you look forward to?*

If some family members look forward to them more than others each family member may be asked of these contacts

- *Who looks forward to them the most?*
- *Who looks forward to them the least?*

Triangles and multigenerational patterns may be identified by first asking questions about alliances. For example, each family member may be asked to point out on the nuclear family part of the genogram

- *Which member of the family is closest to which other member?*

and

- *Which family member is in disagreement with which other member?*

With the Barrows this showed that Sheila and Caroline were involved in a very close relationship and that Dick and Sheila were in disagreement. Together these two pieces of information suggested the presence of what Haley (1967) calls a pathological triangle (which was previously mentioned in Chapter 2). It usually involves a close alliance between a child and a parent and a conflictual relationship between that parent and the other parent. Such triangles are commonly associated with the maintenance of childhood behavioural problems and with psychological symptoms. Often the disagreement concerns the best way to help the child overcome the symptoms.

Multigenerational patterns may be identified by asking about similarities between relationships. For example

- *What relationship in the wider family is most like the relationship between Caroline and Sheila?*

With the Barrows there were clear parallels between Sheila's relationship with her mother and Caroline's relationship with Sheila. This type of mother daughter relationship was also present in the preceding generation.

Karl Tomm (1987a, b, 1988, 1991) gives a thorough account of types of questions that are useful in mapping out patterns of family relationships, belief systems and possibilities for change. The replication of family patterns across generations is an idea that lies at the heart of Murray Bowen's approach to family therapy. A good account of this is given in Friedman (1991).

THE FAMILY LIFECYCLE

While a genogram provides a cross-sectional perspective on family life, the family history provides a longitudinal view of family development. In constructing a family history the therapist is trying to answer the following specific questions. First, how has this family managed the tasks at previous stages of the lifecycle? Second, if difficulties were encountered how were these resolved? Third, how well is it equipped to manage the present stage of the lifecycle, and in particular the current presenting problem? Fourth, why has the family developed problems at this stage in the lifecycle? Thus, the family history is a crucial part of assessment since it throws light on *family coping strategies* and on *precipitating* factors.

The stages of the family lifecycle and associated tasks for the traditional intact family are contained in Figure 6.9. This framework may be used as a basis for interviewing about the family lifecycle. A comprehensive account of the implications of family lifecycle issues for therapeutic practice is given in Carter and McGoldrick's (1989) landmark text. Where separation between family members occurs, additional tasks must be accomplished. I am referring here to tasks associated with divorce, remarriage and fostering. A framework for conceptualising the tasks associated with separation and divorce is presented in Figures 6.10. A more detailed account of lifecycle stages associated with separation is contained in Robinson's (1991) clinical manual. Useful accounts of the special tasks which families must complete in child placement and fostering cases are contained in Thoburn (1988) and Gilligan (1991). The frameworks in Figures 6.9 and 6.10 apply specifically to family life in Westernised cultures, and may be inappropriate for use with other ethnic groups. The likelihood of family members developing symptoms is increased at each of the transition points within the family lifecycle. For example, many referrals in child and family clinics cluster around the transitions associated with the birth of a child, a child's entry into school, the onset of adolescence or a child leaving home. At these transitional times the family is under greater stress than usual.

Two main factors contribute to the stress associated with family lifecycle transitions. The first of these is the number of concurrent tasks that must be completed and the collective demands that these entail. For example, the Barrow family were coping with

STAGE	TASKS
1. Family of origin experiences	* Maintaining relationships with parents, siblings and peers * Completing school
2. Leaving home	* Differentiation of self from family of origin and developing adult to adult relationship with parents * Developing intimate peer relationships * Beginning a career
3. Premarriage stage	* Selecting partners * Developing a relationship * Deciding to marry
4. Childless couple stage	* Developing a way to live together based on reality rather than mutual projection * Realigning relationships with families of origin and peers to include spouses
5. Family with young children	* Adjusting marital system to make space for children * Adopting parenting roles * Realigning relationships with families of origin to include parenting and grandparenting roles
6. Family with adolescents	* Adjusting parent-child relationships to allow adolescents more autonomy * Adjusting marital relationships to focus on midlife marital and career issues * Taking on responsibility of caring for families of origin
7. Launching children	* Negotiating adult to adult relationships with children * Adjusting to living as a couple again * Adjusting to including in-laws and grandchildren within the family circle * Dealing with disabilities and death in the family of origin
8. Later life	* Coping with physiological decline * Adjusting to the children taking a more central role in family maintenance * Making room for the wisdom and experience of the elderly * Dealing with loss of spouse and peers * Preparation for death, life review and integration

Figure 6.9. Stages of the family lifecycle

STAGE	TASK
1. Decision to divorce	* Accepting one's own part in marital failure
2. Planning separation	* Cooperatively developing a plan for custody of the children, visitation and finances * Dealing with the families of origin's response to the plan to separate
3. Separation	* Mourning the loss of the intact family * Adjusting to the change in parent-child and parent-parent relationships * Avoiding letting marital arguments interfere with parent-to- parent cooperation * Staying connected to the extended family * Managing doubts about separation and becoming committed to divorce
4. Post-Divorce period	* Maintaining flexible arrangements about custody, access and finances * Ensuring both parents retain strong relationships with the children * Reestablishing peer relationships and a social network
5. Entering a new relatlonship	* Completing emotional divorce from the previous relationship * Developing commitment to a new marriage
6. Planning a new marriage	* Planning for cooperative co-parental relationships with ex-spouses * Planning to deal with children's loyalty conflicts involving natural and step-parents * Adjust to widening of extended family
7. Establishing a new family	* Realigning relationships within the family to allow space for new members * Sharing memories and histories to allow for integration of all new members

Figure 6.10.   Extra stages in the family lifecycle entailed by separation or divorce and remarriage

having adolescent children, one of whom was ill and one of whom was about to leave home, and also with bereavement, having lost the maternal grandmother in the preceding eighteen months.

The second important factor is the way in which these demands are appraised. The meaning and significance that they hold for the family, and the parents in particular, contributes to the overall impact of lifecycle transitions on the family. Parents' beliefs about the significance of lifecycle transitions and how to manage them are strongly influenced by their experiences of how their issues were dealt with in their families of origin. The beliefs that family members hold about particular issues relevant to lifecycle transitions may help or hinder them in completing developmental tasks effectively. With the Barrows, the beliefs about how to manage children's illnesses, school refusal, leaving home and bereavement held by the parents and based on their own experiences of how these issues were dealt with in their families of origin, were important areas of inquiry in constructing the family history.

The family history constructed by the Barrows showed that Dick had been required to take on a substitute father role in his own family of origin, because his father had left home when he was three years old and his mother subsequently had to spend a lot of time away from the home, working. He adopted a strict, dutiful *no nonsense* approach to managing his brothers, Rex and John who were only one and two years his junior. The family ethos was always one of hard work and duty. When he left school, he got a job in sales. He moved jobs a couple of times but always stayed in the selling field. He met Sheila through his work. They married. He worked long and hard to provide a good house and standard of living for Sheila and the children. She gave up work after Mat was born. Dick had been promoted to area manager status about five years previously, and expected to become a sales director in the next couple of years. He longed for this job in head office because it would mean an end to him having to spend Monday to Friday on the road. However, to get this promotion, he had to supervise his team closely so that they reached their sales targets. This involved him spending five days a week away from the family. From Dick's viewpoint, he and Sheila had always managed all the tasks of family development from marriage through having children, Sheila's miscarriage and her mother's death, with strength and courage.

He saw Caroline's problem as one of disobedience or lack of backbone. When he was asked

- *If your mother was here now, what advice would she give you about how to manage Caroline's problem and would you take it?*

he said that his mother would advise him that Caroline's pains would have to be ignored, and that she should be firmly put to school.

Sheila's family history was quite different. She, as the youngest of three children grew up in a house where both of her parents were always at home in the evenings. She was close to her mother throughout her life. She greatly valued her role as a wife and mother and was quite happy to end her career as a secretary when she did. During her children's early years and during the time following the miscarriage, she obtained a great deal of support from her mother who lived nearby. Dick was very busy at this time and rarely at home. Her mother's cancer was discovered only when she had developed secondary tumours which were inoperable. Sheila still felt guilty about this because on a number of occasions before the cancer was diagnosed, her mother had complained of pain and she had accepted the brush off from her mother's doctor when she had asked him to arrange for investigations.

When I asked her

- *Are you frightened that the doctors may misdiagnose Caroline in the way that they misdiagnosed your Mother?*

Sheila began to cry and said that she feared Caroline had something terrible wrong with her that was being missed. When asked

- *If your mother were here now, what advice would she give you on how to manage Caroline's problem?*

she said that her mother would insist that Caroline's health should be put ahead of all other concerns. A full medical examination should be conducted.

Sheila then spontaneously mentioned that these fears about Caroline's health had coincided with Caroline going back to school in September, the anniversary of her mother's death and the beginning of Mat's last year in secondary school. Next year he would be going away to university and she would miss him deeply. He had been a great support to her in managing practical problems around the house over the years, while Dick was at work. Further inquiry confirmed that Mat had taken on a substitute father role, much like that which Dick had held as a teenager.

ASKING QUESTIONS ABOUT THE FAMILY LIFECYCLE.

The construction of the genogram begins with emotionally neutral questions about demographic characteristics of family members, and ends with emotionally loaded questions about alliances and family patterns. A similar sequence is followed in constructing a family history. Early questions seek factual accounts of events that happened, like leaving home, getting married and the timing of having children, the children going to school and then making the transition to adolescence. Later questions focus on the way in which the parents have internalised the cultures of their families of origin, and the ways in which they bring these assumptions to bear on tackling the tasks associated with lifecycle transitions.

The major pitfalls in constructing a family history are to spend a lot of time and energy on developing an account of events that happened and not enough time on exploring the impact of family-of-origin experiences on the belief systems of the parents.

When inquiring about factual events, it is helpful to use questions that break the lifespan into meaningful temporal chunks and ask about events within these chunks. Here are some such questions.

- *Did any thing unusual happen during your first five years of life?*
- *Was your time at primary school an uneventful period or are there some key events that stand out in your memory?*
- *Between primary school and leaving home, what were the main milestones in your adolescence?*
- *Between leaving home and meeting your spouse, what were the main events in your life?*
- *In your first five years together what things happened that are important markers?*

This type of questioning will usually highlight periods in the lifecycle when the family coped particularly well or poorly with a particular problem. For each of these problem periods it is useful to ask the following sorts of questions.

- *What was the problem?*
- *What sense did each of you make of it?*
- *What different things did you do to get over the problem and who was involved?*
- *If your parents had faced that problem what would they have done?*

These questions will throw light on the ways of looking at problems and beliefs about solving them that parents have, and the extent to which these are based on family-of-origin experiences. Similar sorts of inquiry need to be carried out in relation to the presenting problem. The two critical questions here are

- *How would your mother or father have looked at this problem?*
- *If they were here, what advice would they give you about solving this problem?*

SUMMARY

In Chapter 5 the process of clarifying the cycle of interaction surrounding the presenting problem was described. A description of this pattern of interaction (an example of which is given in Figure 5.2) is placed in the right hand column of the three column formulation model. The beliefs which constrain system members to repeat these behaviour patterns are placed in the central column. The factors which predispose system members to hold these beliefs are placed in the left hand column. These beliefs and the factors on which they are based, may be identified through the process of constructing a history of the referred child's development, a history of the family's development and through the construction of a genogram. Family strengths and protective factors may also be identified during this stage of the assessment. In this chapter frameworks for taking histories and constructing genograms were described. These are based on empirical research findings, useful theoretical frameworks and models of good practice within the field. The importance of distinguishing between developmental events on the one hand and the meaning which family members attribute to these events was a core principle underlying the approach to history taking and genogram construction described here. Significant life events often emerge as important predisposing factors. However, it is the belief systems associated with these that typically link them to repetitive patterns of behaviour which system members engage in when faced with the presenting problem. Pinpointing key features of the histories and the genogram, and integrating these into the three column formulation, is the next step in the assessment process and the focus of Chapter 7.

Exercise 6.1.

Work in pairs.

One person should take the role of interviewer and the other, the role of interviewee.

The interviewer then constructs a family history and genogram with the interviewee using the system described in the chapter.

Swap roles.

Write down
- the three most salient things you noticed about the material produced by the person that you interviewed
- the three main observations you made about the process of interviewing
- the three main things you noticed about being interviewed.

Discuss what you have written down with your partner.

Exercise 6.2.

This exercise is based on the Whitefriar case described in Exercise 4.1.

Work in groups of at least five members. Four people take the roles of family members. The remaining person or people take the roles of the therapist and team.

The therapist (with preconsultation suggestions from the team) constructs

1.   A developmental history
2.   A family history
3.   A genogram.

People role-playing family members need to take 10 minutes to talk together as a family and develop their roles. Therapist and team need to take 10 minutes to plan the way in which the interview will be managed

Take about 30 minutes to role-play the interview.

Derole after the interview.

Take 20 minutes to discuss

1.   What the experience was like for family members.
2.   Which aspects of the interviewing process were within the therapist's competence and which offered the greatest challenge.
3.   The main salient points that emerged for the therapist/team and the family members.

7

Formulation and Contracting for Treatment

KEY ELEMENTS ABSTRACTED FROM THE HISTORY AND GENOGRAM

In constructing the formulation for the Barrow family, we first listed the key points from the developmental and family histories and the genogram before integrating these into a three column formulation, along with the description of the cycle of interaction around the presenting problem (set out in Figure 5.2). These key features were:

1. Sheila's miscarriage

Sheila had a miscarriage prior to conceiving Caroline. Caroline was therefore a highly valued child. The mother-daughter attachment was particularly strong. This replicated the close mother-daughter relationships which characterised Sheila's side of the family for at least the preceding four generations. Sheila was prone to reacting very strongly to any threats to Caroline's well-being.

2. Caroline's gastroenteritis

Caroline had a history of gastroenteritis but was otherwise a healthy teenager with good academic and social skills. She had a strong relationship with her mother, and looked to her for guidance on how to make sense of her predicament. In doing so, she perceived her mother's anxiety about her health. Consequently she believed herself to have some undiagnosed illness.

3. Grandmother's undiagnosed cancer

Sheila had lost her mother exactly a year prior to the onset of Caroline's abdominal pain and school-refusal. She felt guilty for not insisting that the physician examine her mother earlier. If this had happened, then the maternal grandmother might not have developed secondaries and an early operation could have prolonged her life. Sheila believed that she might be involved in a similar situation with Caroline, where some important illness was being missed by the involved medical personnel.

4. Sheila's use of health as a core construct

Sheila construed Caroline's difficulty as primarily a health problem, because in her family of origin, health was a core construct for making sense of the world and was valued above all else.

5. Sheila's cognitive style

Like her mother, who suffered recurrent depression, Sheila was prone to maximising the negative and minimising the positive. In this context, she was prone to attending to signs of Caroline's ill-health selectively and to disregarding or minimising her signs of well-being.

6. Dick's use of duty and discipline as core constructs

Dick had grown up in a family where he took on a paternal role at an early age. He brought up his two brothers after his father had deserted the family when Dick was three years old. During this time he developed a set of values, under the influence of his mother who was a hard worker, that served him well in this difficult role. He took a rigid, dutiful, no-nonsense approach to child rearing. Obedience to authority was highly valued by him. Duty and discipline were core constructs in the way his family made sense of the world. Illness, and other forms of vulnerability were denied or minimised. He therefore interpreted Caroline's predicament as essentially a discipline problem, a failure to do one's duty.

7. Dick's career path

Dick desperately wanted to be promoted into a position where he would not have to spend time away from home in the long term. He believed that to attain this promotion he must spend a lot of time away from home in the short term. Hence, his absence from family life.

8. Mat's need to leave home

Mat identified with his father's worldview and saw the family difficulties as a discipline problem. However, his main concern was finishing school and going to college, so he did not want to become too involved in the battle between Caroline and Sheila.

9. Multigenerational history of close mother-daughter relationships

Going back four generations, the women on Sheila's side of the family had always had close mother-daughter relationships. Thus Caroline and her mother found themselves unquestioningly in a very close and intimate type of relationship where mutual emotional influence was particularly strong.

10. Caroline's social support network

For Caroline, Kirsty, her close friend could neutralize the impact of her mother's anxiety about her. She could help Caroline believe that it was only a transient discomfort and could direct Caroline's attention to other issues.

11. Sheila's social support network

For Sheila, contact with her friend Mary, the GP, or Dick, lessened her anxiety about Caroline. She felt supported by them and this lessened her belief that she would be responsible for a catastrophe where Caroline's illness would go undiagnosed.

LINKING THE ELEMENTS TO THE FORMULATION

The next step in constructing the formulation was to link these key elements abstracted for the histories and genogram to the cycle of interaction surrounding the problem. Our formulation is presented in Figure 7.1.

The formulation shows how the specific beliefs of each family member constrain them to act as they do during an episode of the problem. Furthermore, these beliefs are linked to predisposing factors such as stressful life events or early socialization experiences in the family of origin.

CONSTRUCTION AND PRESENTATION OF THE FORMULATION

There are many useful ways of organising the construction and presentation of the formulation. In Positive Practice, the standard approach is for the therapist to take a break once the assessment procedures have been completed. Then, in a brief fifteen or twenty minute recess, the formulation is constructed. The treatment implications of the formulation or the objectives of further assessment are specified. The therapist then presents the formulation and its implications to the family, and offers a contract for further consultation to follow through on the implications of the formulation.

With the Barrows, I took a break for twenty minutes and sketched out the hypothesis on a flipchart page. I also gave some thought to the implications of this for further consultation. Future therapy in this case would have to focus on the parents developing a unified way of making sense of the problem and dealing with it. I thought it might also require the involvement of school personnel in the management plan.

In addition to presenting the formulation and offering a contract for therapy, I wanted to give all family members a sense that they had been understood and that there was hope that the problem could be resolved. Empathy and the generation of hope are important aspects of all good therapeutic practice (Frank,1967). Here is how the formulation was presented and the contract for further work offered.

Therapist: I have been piecing together all the parts of this problem..eh..as I see it now. It's a complex situation.....a tough problem .....but I think....I'm certain that there is a solution. That's the first thing I want to say. I think there is a way of understanding the problem that points to a solution. So let's look at this diagram first. You recognise this bit here? (pointing to right hand column).

Dick: mmmm.

Therapist: This is a typical episode from the time Sheila: wakes up in the morning till Dick calls at night. Now what I've tried to do is guess from all the other things

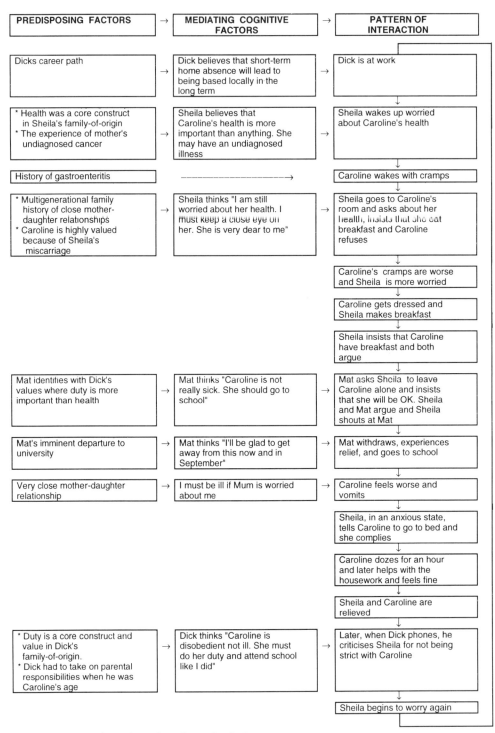

Figure 7.1.   A three column formulation for the Barrow case

you've said to me what forces you to repeat this dance again and again one week after another for months. That's the question. How is it that this keeps repeating? I mean .....that's the mystery.

Sheila: Yes. I know......She might be...But she is.. she might be very ill.

Therapist: (to Sheila) Well Caroline..... my opinion is....she's in a lot of pain nearly every morning. Real pain. Now maybe it doesn't show up on an X-ray but then neither does a headache or a migraine. And we all know that they are real pain. ....eh ...Bad pain. You know we all have our Achilles heel. Some people get headaches when they get sick and some people get pains in their joints. But Caroline, we know that your Achilles heel is in your stomach. When you get run down, you get a bad stomach. So where does that leave us? Oh yes...I want to point out that I've included Caroline's vulnerability to stomach problems...her Achilles heel..... here on the map of the problem (points to third listed predisposing factor).

Caroline: Yes. m.. hm

Therapist: (to Sheila) Well Sheila:... when you wake up, you go and check on Caroline because you know she gets a bad stomach. My guess is that you don't want the thing that happened with your mum to happen again. And in your family health was a central concern. You said to me that your mum said "Your health is the main thing." So that's the way you think about Caroline. Are you with me so far? (Sheila nods.) The other thing is, you are really close to your daughter so you sense what she feels and she feels what you feel ..eh.. what concerns you. That's the way all the mothers and daughters have done things in your family going back four generations as far as I understand it?

Sheila: Yes my mother.... She and I were just like that.

Therapist: And she was like that with her mother, you said..you said earlier?

Sheila: Yes that's right.

Therapist: So I've put those things: the concern with health in your family, the unfortunate situation with your mother's diagnosis and the special kind of relationships mums and daughters have in your family in here (points to the relevant predisposing factors).

Sheila: Yes. I see.

Therapist: (to Sheila:) These are my best guess at what you say to yourself in these situations....sort of simplifications of what you might say. Not exactly what you say.. but the gist of what you think to yourself privately. Do they hit the spot?

Sheila: Well. .....Yes sometimes I think ...eh... She's getting worse.

Therapist: (to Caroline) And I'm guessing that you think to yourself.......this sort of thing...(Points to "I must be ill if Mum is worried about me." part of the formulation diagram.)

Caroline: Not really...

Therapist: You don't think that at the front of your mind? But I'm guessing that you see mum being worried and maybe this is at the back of your mind..maybe even in your unconscious...I'm not sure....but I think so?

Caroline: mmm...

Therapist: (to Dick). You talked about short term sacrifice for long term gain. I put that in here (indicates place in formulation). You also talked about the importance of duty in your family when you brought your brothers up and how you see Caroline's school absence as ...eh....not doing what is expected of her. So .....that is in the map too just here. When you phone Sheila you say Caroline must not get away with this....Like she is disobedient...and your wife says ..."But she is sick" ...That's the main conflict between you about this whole thing ....two ways of looking at the same thing ...I suppose ..two very different constructions.

Dick: Yes she must do what she is told. If her mother tells her to go to school, she must go.

Therapist: You have strong views about this, Dick, so they are included in the map. Now, Mat, I guess you share Dad's view so I put that in here (indicates Mat's position). I also suspect you want to be freed up a bit from this situation to, eh... to do what you need to do next ...in college and that.

Mat: Yea.....that's it.

Therapist: So what this map is saying is...your beliefs are tying you all into this circle and your beliefs are rooted in where each of you has come from. Important things that have happened in the past....or are going on now outside the family. Can you accept this map as a rough description of the problem you have brought here? Not the truth...just a *good enough* map.

Dick: Yes. In a nutshell....yes ...you put it in a nutshell there.

Sheila: Yes but she..Caroline.. is ill.

Therapist: That is included in the picture Sheila (points to predisposing factor of gastroenteritis history).

Caroline: Can you accept it?

Sheila: Yes.

Therapist: Well. It follows from this that there are some things that can be done to solve the problem. Would you be interested in hearing about those things now?

Dick: Yes. that's what we're here for.

Caroline and Sheila: Yes.

At this point it was suggested that the objective of further consultations would be to help the parents find a way of developing a plan to work together to help Caroline deal with the pain and return to school, even though they held very different beliefs about the nature of the problem. This broad objective was accepted and the process of setting specific goals was deferred until the next appointment.

A contract for six further sessions was offered: three within office hours and three outside office hours to accommodate Dick's working arrangements. The contract was accepted by each of the family members.

Sheila and Dick were offered the task of discussing the various courses of action that would follow from their different beliefs about the problem and to list the pros and cons associated with each course of action.

Caroline was invited to record a pain rating three times a day on a ten point scale, and to note factors that effected the intensity of these ratings.

Mat was invited to withdraw from further involvement in the problem altogether.

That concluded the intake interview with the Barrows. A checklist that itemizes the sequence of events to follow when presenting a formulation and offering a contract for therapy is contained in Figure 7.2. The process of reading the referral letters, contracting for assessment, conducting the assessment interview, constructing the formulation and presenting this to the family, along with a contract for therapy, took about two hours.

FEEDBACK CHECKLIST

1. Generate hope by defining the problem as solvable
2. Empathise with each person's position as you explain the formulation
3. Check that the formulation has been accepted
4. Suggest an overall objective for further consultation
5. Offer a flexible contract for therapy
6. Invite family members to do assessment related tasks
7. Set the next appointment

Figure 7.2. Checklist for the feedback section of the intake interview

STRUCTURING THE INTAKE INTERVIEW

The way in which the intake interview with the Barrows was structured follows in the tradition of the original Milan group (Selvini-Palazzoli et al, 1978b) who formalized the five part session. In the first part the team would meet to develop a plan. In the second the interview would be conducted by one member of the team and observed by the other three. In the third the team would hold a meeting separate from the family. Here a systemic hypothesis would be developed and a message or intervention for the family developed. In the fourth part of the interview this would be delivered to the family. The fifth part of the session was reserved for reflecting on the family's response to the message or intervention.

The structure of the Barrows' intake interview also shares much in common with the medical tradition and the practice of behaviour therapy. Within each of these traditions it is also routine practice to gather information with the client and then to integrate this into a coherent formulation in privacy before rejoining the patient and advising on plans for further assessment or therapy. In many circumstances, particularly if the therapist or team find the case anxiety provoking, it may be useful to formulate the case in privacy. This will facilitate anxiety reduction and clear thinking. Anxiety provoking situations include being a novice and handling a case unsupervised; being experienced but managing a complex multiproblem case; or dealing with a case that triggers strong countertransference reactions because it resonates with unresolved personal issues (Carr, 1989).

However, there are other ways of structuring the session so that the family may either observe or participate more fully in the formulation process. Within the family therapy field Andersen's (1987) reflecting team is one of the most influential innovations in this area. Here, the family observe the team through a one-way screen as they sift through the assessment information and reach a formulation or hypothesis during the midsession break. Active-interactional cotherapy is another innovation that allows the family an opportunity to observe formulation construction (Hoffman and Gafni, 1984). Here a pair of cotherapists discuss their differing viewpoints from time to time during the course of the sessions, thus allowing the family an opportunity to observe ideas about the problem being formulated by the cotherapy team. A third approach to practice in this area is for the therapist to co-construct the formulation with the help of the family within the therapy session. With this approach, at various points in the session, the therapist fills in different sections of the three column formulation with the help of the family on a whiteboard or flipchart in the consulting room. This highly participative session structure is the approach that I use most frequently at present. It has the advantage of increasing family members' sense of participation in therapy and therefore their commitment to change (Carr, 1990c). However it also carries disadvantages. It increases the likelihood that the therapist through the development of countertransference reactions will inadvertently become sucked into patterns of interaction with the family that prevent rather than promote problem resolution (Carr, 1989).

Positive Practice requires the therapist to weigh up both of these factors before deciding on how best to manage this stage of the intake interview. The family therapy field is divided over how best to manage this dilemma. What follows is a brief account of how the two camps deal with this set of issues, and the implications of each position for Positive Practice.

THE IMPLICATIONS OF STRUCTURALISM AND SOCIAL CONSTRUCTIVISM FOR POSITIVE PRACTICE

The use of a team, a screen, and veiling the formulation process in secrecy, derives from a collection of theoretical positions which include first order cybernetics and structuralism (Guttman, 1991). These positions hold in common the view that dysfunctional family structures give rise to symptomatic behaviour in one or more family members. The team behind the screen are in a position to observe the structural aberrations within the referred family and to plan ways in which these may be changed. Therapy conducted from this type of model construes the relationship between the family and the therapeutic team in adversarial terms, and military metaphors are commonly used to describe the team's activities. Strategy, tactics, resistance, intervention, structural change and dirty games are terms drawn from the vocabulary of this family therapy tradition. The tradition includes strategic (Madanes, 1991) and structural (Colapinto, 1991) family therapy models along with those developed by Selvini-Palazzoli's current group (Selvini-Palazzoli et al, 1989).

The use of reflecting teams, active interactional cotherapy and an open cooperative approach to formulation, characterises a contrasting tradition within the family therapy field. The tradition looks to the second order cybernetics of observing systems, to social-constructionism, the narrative tradition, and to post-modernism for its theoretical roots (Hoffman, 1990; McNamee and Gergen, 1991). The cybernetics of observing systems entails the view that the problem creates the system rather than that the system creates the problem (Anderson et al, 1986). That is, when a family, a professional network and a therapist come together to solve a problem they organise themselves into a system. On some occasions this system may repeatedly fail to solve the presenting problem, or indeed compound it. This is quite different from the structuralist view that the dysfunctional system creates the problem. The narrative tradition emphasises the idea that the problem-determined system is constructed through language. Social constructionism and post-modernism entail the view that problems, solutions, and other concepts are not independently existing objective realities to be discovered. They are, rather, meanings which are coconstructed by therapists and clients and brought forth in therapeutic conversations. From this perspective the task of the therapist is to host a therapeutic conversation where a new and more useful way of construing the problem will emerge that will facilitate problem resolution. Therapy conducted from this perspective is a collaborative and participative venture. Conversation, discourse, narrative and curiosity are common metaphors used to characterise the therapeutic relationship. The therapist is curious about the client's unfortunate story and helps the client edit this to develop a more useful narrative, rather than assessing resistance and developing a strategy for change. The tradition includes among others Boscolo and Cecchin in Italy, Hoffman, Penn and Anderson in the US, Draper and Campbell in the UK and McCarthy, Byrne and Kearney in Ireland (Campbell et al, 1991; Kenny, 1988).

In Positive Practice useful elements of both the structural and social-constructionist traditions must be identified and integrated. Let us take the example of conduct disorders. That is, youngsters who become involved in adversarial and antisocial relationships with others. A large body of empirical evidence indicates that certain reliably identifiable structural characteristics of social systems predispose youngsters to acquire a DSM-IV diagnosis of conduct disorder (APA, 1994). These risk factors include: poverty, maternal depression, paternal deviance or absence, a chaotic family lifestyle, learning difficulties and membership of a poorly organized school (Kazdin, 1991). No therapeutic conversation can reedit the significance of these risk factors. In Positive Practice clinicians need to identify such structural factors in their assessment, and include these risk factors in their formulation, particularly in cases where abuse, violence or suicide are suspected. In this way the structural tradition contributes to Positive Practice.

Let us now take an example where the ideas drawn from the second cybernetics of observing systems offers a particularly useful lens through which to view a difficult clinical problem. A therapist who only offered appointments within office hours complained that the father of a family he was seeing rarely attended therapy. The therapist attributed the poor progress the case was making to the low level of the father's involvement in the consultation process. He described the family as resistant, as if the resistance was a structural quality of the family, rather than a characteristic of the problem-system of which he was part. When we discussed the difficulty from an observing system's perspective, the therapist began to see how he was contributing to the resistance which he was attributing to the family. He subsequently rescheduled some appointments to include the father outside of office hours and arranged for sessions with other family members to focus on issues other than the father's *resistance* to change.

Positive Practice rests on the cornerstone of social-constructionism. In every case, regardless of the risk factors and structural constraints, there is room for a therapist to construct with the client a new and different way of construing the client's dilemma or problem which is more useful. That is, every session is an opportunity for the therapist and client to hold a conversation about the problem in a way that opens up new options and possibilities for problem resolution. Selective attention, therapeutic creativity, the ambiguity of social and community living, and the characteristics of language are among the more important factors that make this possible. This issue will be taken up again when reframing and relabelling are discussed as important therapeutic measures in the middle phase of therapy in Chapter 10.

SUMMARY

In Chapter 6, history taking and genogram construction were described. These assessment procedures generate a wealth of information from which the clinician must distil a number of key features that have relevance to the construction of a useful formulation. In this chapter we reviewed how these key pieces of information, drawn from history taking and genogram construction, may be integrated into the three column formulation model. We then looked at different clinical methods for carrying out this process and presenting the formulation to the family. One of the alternatives is to construct the formulation in privacy and to present it to clients in its finished state. Another is to coconstruct the formulation with the family. Between these two extremes are the options of using a reflecting teams approach or engaging in active interactional cotherapy.

The implications of two contrasting theoretical positions: structuralism and social-constructionism for Positive Practice were also discussed. We then looked at the way in which the presentation of the formulation and the family's acceptance of it provides a basis for offering a contract for further consultation. The importance of empathy and hope were highlighted. In our case example, each family member was invited to carry out a simple task between the first and second sessions and implicit therapeutic goals were set. Inviting family members to carry out tasks between sessions, and making implicit therapeutic goals explicit, are crucial skills in Positive Practice. These skills provide a focus for the next two chapters.

Exercise 7.1

This exercise is based on the Whitefriar case described in Exercise 4.1.

Work in groups of at least five members. Four people take the roles of family members. The remaining person or people take the roles of the therapist and team.

The therapist and team construct a three column formulation which integrates the salient points from the history and genogram identified in Exercise 6.2 with the pattern of interaction around the presenting problem constructed in Exercise 5.1.

The therapist then presents the formulation to the family .

People role-playing family members need to take 10 minutes to talk together as a family and to develop their roles. Therapist and team need to take 10 minutes to plan the way in which the interview will be managed.

Take about 30 minutes to role-play the interview.

Derole after the interview.

Take 20 minutes to discuss

1.   What the experience was like for family members
2.   Which aspects of the interviewing process were within the therapist's competence which offered the greatest challenge.

8

Goals

With the Barrow family the contract for further therapy which was offered entailed an implicit overall goal: that of helping the family break free from the repetitive cycle of interaction which surrounded the presenting problem. In Positive Practice this is always the central goal of consultation: empowering the members of the problem-system to liberate themselves from the cycle in the right hand column of the three column formulation model. For the Barrows, this implicit superordinate goal entailed a number of possible implicit subgoals. These included:

1. That Caroline get rid of the pain.
2. That Caroline return to school.
3. That Sheila , Dick, Caroline and the school staff develop a co-ordinated approach to managing the problem.
4. That Sheila , Dick, Caroline and the school staff evolve a shared understanding of the problem.

At the close of the first session, these subgoals were fairly clear to me. However, I postponed any discussion of them because explicit goal setting, if the family are to own and work towards the goals, takes a lot of time. We were all tired, so I deferred goal setting until the second session.

It was my intention to review how the Barrows handled the tasks that were given in the first part of the second session and then, in the light of their response to the tasks and the review of these, help each family member to articulate explicit therapeutic goals. In this chapter, guidelines for goal setting in Positive Practice will be given. The controversy over the place of goal setting in family therapy will also be discussed.

GOAL SETTING IN POSITIVE PRACTICE

Goal setting is a process whereby the therapist offers clients an opportunity to explore and articulate how they would like things to work out, should therapy be successful. Goal setting in Positive Practice is helpful if certain conditions are met. These conditions are based on my own clinical experience and on a review of the empirical literature on goal setting in a variety of clinical and non-clinical contexts (Carr, 1993). First, family members must articulate clear, specific goals. Second, family members are more likely to complete therapeutic tasks that lead to moderately challenging goals, rather than goals that are unrealistically difficult to achieve or too easy to reach. The degree to which clients construe goals as challenging will depend both upon their abilities and skills on the one hand, and their self-confidence in using these skills on the other. Third, family members must be committed to attaining the goals they set. That is, they must accept the goals and have a personal stake in attaining them. For goals to be accepted they must be consistent with family members' beliefs and values. This includes both beliefs and values held by individual family members and those shared by the family as a whole. Fourth, in family consultation, individual and family goals must be compatible. Fifth, when goal attainment is explicitly assessed periodically, goals are pursued more diligently. Let us now explore each of these conditions for effective goal setting in more detail, by framing them as guidelines for Positive Practice and by making reference to case examples.

1. Help clients to set specific, concrete, visualizable goals

Asking clients to visualise in concrete detail precisely how they would go about their day to day activities if the problem were solved is a particularly effective way of helping clients to articulate therapeutic goals. Here are some typical examples.

- *Imagine, its a year from now and the problem is solved. Its a Monday morning at your house. What is happening? Give me a blow-by-blow description of what everyone is doing.*
- *Suppose your difficulties were sorted out and someone sneaked into your house and made a video of you all going about your business as usual. What would we all see if we watched this videotape?*
- *If there were a miracle tomorrow and your problem was solved, what would be happening in your life.*

This last question, which owes its origin to Milton Erickson, plays a central role in deShazer's solution-focused approach to therapy. He refers to it as the *Miracle Question*. Indeed, deShazer found that the clarity with which clients answered this question was the single best predictor of therapeutic outcome (Carr, 1990e).

Questions which ask the client to visualise some intermediate step along the road to problem resolution, may help clients to elaborate intermediate goals or to clarify the endpoint at which they are aiming. Here are some questions that fall into this category.

- *Mary, just say this problem was half-way better. What would you notice different about the way your mum and dad and brother talked to each other?*
- *What would be the difference between the way you argue now and the way you would argue if you were half-way down the road to solving this difficulty?*

The following set of goal setting questions involves asking clients about the minimum degree of change that would need to occur for them to believe that they had begun the journey down the road to problem resolution.

- *What is the first thing I would notice if I walked into your house if things were just beginning to change for the better?*
- *What is the smallest thing that would have to change for you to know you were moving in the right direction to solve this difficult problem?*

The MRI group ask clients to set these minimal changes as their therapeutic goals. They believe that once these small changes occur and are perceived, a snowball effect takes place, and the positive changes become more and more amplified without further therapeutic intervention (Segal, 1991). In Positive Practice, these minimal goals are set, where the therapist must work under severe time constraints or where clients have had their self-confidence in their problem-solving skills seriously depleted through repeated failures.

2. Help clients to set moderately challenging goals which take account of both clients' abilities and skills on the one hand and their self-confidence in using these talents on the other

In Positive Practice therapists may base their expert judgements of the appropriateness of clients' goals on a variety of factors, including direct observation, test results, outside reports, second opinions and their knowledge of the relevant scientific and clinical literature. Let us look at these bases for making judgements about the appropriateness of clients' goals in more detail.

Judgements about goals may derive from direct observation of clients performing tasks in the intake session. For example, with a parent-teenager communication problem, I asked the father and son to reach agreement on how late the youngster could stay out on midsummer's night. This showed me that both family members, who had very low confidence in their ability to communicate, were capable of stating their positions clearly, but had poor listening skills. Fortunately these were skills that could be improved with coaching.

The therapist may also base his judgement of ability and skill levels on the results of tests or school reports. An eleven year old boy and his mother came for a consultation because of the boy's supposed laziness and inattentiveness at school. The mother's implicit goal was to help her son to overcome his laziness. He had been middle of his class in primary school but when he went up to secondary school he failed his term exams. A brief psychometric evaluation of the boy's basic academic skills and intelligence showed that his attainment and ability levels all fell well below the normal range. There was no doubt from the school report that the boy had become demoralised and lazy about his school work, probably because the curriculum and the pace of teaching were not geared to his ability level. These factors were taken into account when setting goals in this case.

In Positive Practice the therapist also bases expert judgement of clients' potential skills and abilities on knowledge of the relevant scientific and clinical literature. This is particularly important where referred children have paediatric conditions such as asthma, diabetes and epilepsy, or disabilities such as visual impairment or mental handicap. Parents, teachers or other involved professionals may have unrealistic expectations of the sorts of goals that youngsters may achieve. In some cases the problem is one of overestimation. The parents of a child with ME (myalgic encephalomylitis) who had been housebound for a month, expected that, with appropriate guidance, he would return to normal activity levels within a fortnight. As part of goal setting, the family were informed that a realistic recovery time for this condition runs to months rather than weeks.

In other cases, the resourcefulness of the youngster may be underestimated. The parents of a diabetic teenager, referred for depression, continually thwarted all of the girl's attempts at developing autonomy and self-sufficiency, because they saw her condition as dangerous and extremely disabling and feared she might be incapable of managing her illness and her life. The girl had come to accept this view of herself as vulnerable, dependent and incapable of independence by the time the referral for consultation was made. As part of the goal setting process we told the girl and her parents about other diabetic teenagers who, despite the illness, developed autonomy and independence in much the same way as youngsters without the condition.

Where there is doubt about the constraints imposed by certain conditions with which clients present, it is Positive Practice to refer the case to a colleague for a second opinion or an expert assessment. This expert opinion is then included in the goal setting process.

This very obvious point needs to be made because of a dangerous trend in the field of family therapy. There is a hazardous tendency within the field for Gurus to emerge and unwittingly give the message to new practitioners that a competent clinician should be able to manage cases either alone or within the confines of a family therapy team (L'Abate and Jurkovic, 1987). Of course it is more honest and ethical to accept that we are all bounded by the knowledge limits imposed on us by our discipline, our clinical experience and our reading. It is not useful for clinicians to expect themselves to have a comprehensive knowledge of paediatric, psychiatric, psychological, educational, occupational social and legal implications of the problems of all referred cases. In Positive Practice, when in doubt about these issues, a second opinion is sought.

3. Explore the costs and benefits of goals

A variety of future scenarios, possibilities and goals will be explored in most cases. The costs and benefits of these may usefully be explored using a variety of questioning styles. Circular questions about gains and losses are a particularly effective way of conducting this exploration. Here are some examples from the Barrow case.

- *Mat, what do you think your mother and sister would lose from their relationship if Caroline recovered?*
- *Dick, what do you think Sheila would miss most from your telephone conversations if Caroline were better now?*
- *Dick, if Caroline recovered, what do you think she and Sheila would lose from their relationship?*
- *Sheila, what do you believe Dick would gain if you all worked towards Caroline's recovery, and what would be the price that he would have to pay?*

- *Mat—of your mum, your dad and Caroline—who would face the most hassles if they all worked towards Caroline's recovery?*

Circular questions are particularly useful for making explicit, implicit beliefs that family members hold that are relevant to goal attainment. Where direct questions lead to puzzlement, denial of benefits associated with problems and hassles associated with the process of goal attainment, circular questions provide a wealth of information about family beliefs. Circular questions capitalise upon people's capacity to observe others closely and to infer what they may be thinking and their willingness to do so. The problem with direct questions is that people are often unaware of the benefits of their actions or the hidden costs of seemingly reasonable alternative courses of action. However, once circular questions have made implicit beliefs or possibilities explicit, direct questions have an important role to play in establishing whether family members accept goals and are committed to them.

4. Do not explore ways of reaching goals until it is clear that clients accept and are committed to them

After a detailed exploration of the costs and benefits of various goals, clients' acceptance of one set of goals and their commitment to them needs to be clarified. Two key direct questions may be asked to check for acceptance and commitment.

- *Do you want to work towards these goals?*
- *Are you prepared to accept the losses and hassles that go with accepting and working towards these goals?*

If clients say that they want to work towards the goals, this indicates that they have probably accepted them. However, the crucial thing is whether or not they are committed to pursuing them. The second question addresses this issue by asking clients to consider if they can give up the valuable experiences that are entailed by living with a difficult problem. For example, in the Barrow case, Caroline's symptoms provided a forum for both Caroline and her mother to experience an intense sense of emotional attachment to each other. It also provided Dick with a focus for the emotional pain that goes with being an estranged father and a way for him to remain connected to family life while on the road. He would feel duty bound to call regularly to check with his wife how she and Caroline were managing. The second question also tackles the issues of commitment by asking clients if they are prepared to take on all the hassles that go with working towards goals. These hassles include breaking routines, dealing with emotionally painful situations, regular attendance for consultations, and completing homework assignments between sessions. When clients have discussed these factors and say that they are prepared to accept these hassles to get the benefit of achieving their goals, then they are probably committed to the goals they have set.

If clients cannot address the acceptance and commitment questions positively, then goal attainment is unlikely. The following example illustrates this point.

A single mother with a non-compliant six year old was referred by a concerned GP for therapy. During the intake interview the mother said that she and her son had about seven or eight big fights a day. The mother agreed to an initial goal of reducing the fights to no more than four per day. But when she was asked to explore the emotional costs of helping her son develop temper control skills, she balked at the idea that things might get worse before any improvement occurred. She was reluctant to attend regular consultations. She accepted the goals of therapy but she could not make a commitment to them.

5. Help family members construct personal goals and overall family goals that are compatible

One of the major challenges in family therapy is to evolve a construction of the presenting problems that opens up possibilities where each family member's wishes and needs may be respected, when these different needs and wishes are apparently conflicting. Helping family members to articulate the differences and similarities between their positions in considerable detail, and inviting them to explore goals to which they can both agree, first, is a useful method of practice here.

Polly, a fifteen year old girl referred because of school difficulties said that she wanted to be independent. Her parents wanted her to be obedient. Both wanted to be able to live together without continuous hassle. Detailed questioning about what would be happening if Polly to were independent and obedient revealed that both Polly and her parents wanted her to be able, among other things, to speak French fluently. This would help Polly achieve her personal goal of working in France as an *au pair* and would satisfy the parents' goal of her obediently doing school work. Getting a passing grade in French in the term exam was set as a therapy goal. It reflected the family goal of reducing hassle and the individual goals of Polly and her parents.

6. Regularly review progress towards goals

Ideally progress towards goals should be assessed in an observable way or in a quantitative manner. For many problems, progress may be assessed using frequency counts, for example, the number of fights, the number of wet beds, the number of compliments, the number of successes. Ratings of internal states are useful ways of quantifying progress towards less observable goals. Here are some examples of scaling questions.

- *You say that on a scale of one to ten your mood is now about 3. How many points would it have to go up the scale for you to know you were beginning to recover?*
- *If you were recovered, where would your mood be on a 10 point scale most days?*
- *Look at this line. One end stands for how you felt after the car accident. The other, for the feeling of elation you had when you were told about your promotion.*

Low mood after car accident		High mood after promotion

- *Can you show me where you are on that line now and where you want to be when you have found a way to deal with your condition?*

Both solution focused-therapists (deShazer, 1988) and behaviour therapists (Falloon, 1991) commonly use rating scales, but for different reasons. Solution-focused therapists, working within a constructivist framework, use scaling questions to help clients construct a version of the problem that allows the client to perceive personal progress. Behaviour therapists work within a positivist empirical tradition and use rating scales (or frequency counts) to assess what they describe as the objective effectiveness of their interventions. If no change occurs on the scales, then it is the therapist's responsibility to design more effective interventions to help the client reach the agreed goals.

Where clients have difficulty in identifying behaviours that can be counted, or internal states that can be rated using scales, images and metaphors may be used as a way of charting change. A fourteen year old boy was referred with depression following a self-injurious gesture. The depression was associated with frequent changes in residence necessitated by his father's military career. The boy's confession of extreme unhappiness and the episode of self-destructive behaviour came as a shock to his parents because to them his behaviour was as it had always been. Helping the boy to improve his mood was identified as the goal of therapy. The parents could not identify any behavioural changes that would demonstrate that therapeutic progress was being made. The boy said that he could not describe profound mood changes through reference to trivial scales. After much exploration, he evolved a metaphor for his mood state based on a landscape scene in a gothic fantasy novel he was reading. This complex landscape included treacherous mountains, low dark, lightening filled clouds, a dangerous forest and an area of desert. The landscape was inhabited by a variety of mystical creatures and by two tribes representing the forces of good and evil. He was able to visualise this landscape as it was in a period of plague and also as it might be when the dark forces had been defeated. The metaphor of the landscape became the scale through which therapeutic progress was charted. Coincidentally, the regular process of inquiring about the landscape provided his parents with an avenue through which to develop a less authoritarian relationship with their son, one in which they would listen to and take on board his viewpoint.

In Positive Practice all clients are helped to develop some quantitative way for reviewing change towards or away from specific goals. Feedback from periodic review helps the therapist and the clients in two ways. If the feedback is positive, it helps the clients develop self-confidence in their abilities to solve problems and to make progress, and this self-confidence empowers them to tackle other aspects of the solution (Bandura, 1981). If a review of progress towards goals is negative, it provides the therapist and the client with the vital information that they need to change the way that they are trying to solve the presenting problem.

In Positive Practice the therapeutic contract always includes some statement about goal attainment and an episode of therapy is completed when these goals have been reached. For example, if a child is referred for encopresis, the contract may be to help the child complete a two week stretch without soiling his underwear.

Incidentally, the approach to consultation taken in Positive Practice often leads to other positive effects besides removing symptoms. For example, relationships may improve or family members may understand their difficulties better. However, the first episode of treatment usually centres on the child's symptoms and their management. If clients wish to pursue other therapeutic avenues in a second episode of consultation then this is postponed until the first episode is completed. These issues are discussed more fully in Chapters 1 and 16.

GOAL SETTING IN POSITIVE PRACTICE

1.	Help clients to set specific, visualizable goals
2.	Help clients to set moderately challenging goals which take account of both clients' skills and their self-confidence in using these talents
3.	Explore the costs and benefits of goals
4.	Do not explore ways of reaching goals until it is clear that clients accept and are committed to these
5.	Help family members construct personal goals and overall family goals that are compatible
6.	Regularly review progress towards goals

Figure 8.1   Guidelines for setting goals

SUMMARY

After assessment, when a contract for therapy is being offered, an important part of this process is goal setting. In Positive Practice the central goal of consultation is always to empower the members of the problem-system to liberate themselves from the repetitive cycle of interaction which surrounds the presenting problem: the cycle described in the right hand column of the three column formulation model. Clients are helped to develop specific, concrete, visualizable goals. These must be moderately challenging and must take account of clients skills and abilities on the one hand and their confidence in these talents on the other. In Positive Practice therapists may base their expert judgements of the appropriateness of clients' goals on a variety of factors, including direct observation, test results, outside reports, second opinions and their knowledge of the relevant scientific and clinical literature. The pros and cons of various sets of goals need to be examined before identifying one set of goals to work towards. A major pitfall in goal directed therapy occurs when therapists begin to help clients work towards goals before offering clients the space to confirm their acceptance of the therapeutic goals and their commitment to them. In Positive Practice, the therapist never assumes that clients want to work for a set of goals until they have explicitly stated their acceptance of the goals, and have carried out sufficient exploration of the costs of pursuing these goals to be able to make an informed commitment to them. A unique challenge in working with families and wider systems is developing sets of personal and family goals that complement each other, particularly when it appears that families and individuals have conflicting interests. In Positive Practice, goals are reviewed regularly. Frequency counts of symptoms or behaviours, ratings of moods or internal states, and metaphors which represent the presenting problem are useful tools for tracking changes in aspects of the problem over the course of consultation. Tracking progress is important in Positive Practice because knowledge of positive changes enhances clients' self-confidence, and negative feedback allows the therapist and the clients to explore different ways of pursuing therapeutic goals.

Exercise 8.1.

Paul Stuart (whom we first met in Chapter 4) is aged nine and was referred by the GP who identified encopresis, attainment problems and disobedience at home as the main problems. He attended the first session with his mother and two older brothers, and the second session with all family members. The three column formulation set out in Figure 8.2 was constructed and presented to the family. They have accepted it.

Work in groups of at least 6 members. Five people take the roles of family members. The remaining person or people take the roles of the therapist and team.

The therapist and team develop a plan for setting two goals with the Stuart family, following the guidelines set out in this chapter.

People role-playing family members need to take 10 minutes to talk together as a family and develop their roles. Therapist and team need to take 10 minutes to plan the way in which the interview will be managed.

Take about 30 minutes to role-play the interview.

Derole after the interview.

Take 20 minutes to discuss

1.   What the experience was like for family members
2.   Which aspects of the interviewing process were within the therapist's competence and which offered the greatest challenge.

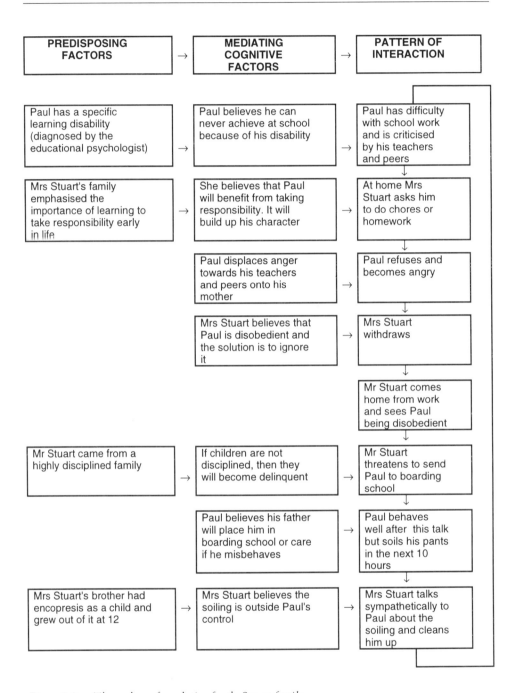

Figure 8.2.   Three column formulation for the Stuart family

9

Tasks between Sessions

Clients may be invited to carry out tasks both within therapy sessions and between sessions. Here our concern is with intersession tasks. A discussion of insession tasks will be reserved for Chapter 10. Family members may be assigned tasks between sessions both to *assess* how the problem-system functions and to empower clients to *change* the problem-system. That is to say, tasks may be used to test hypotheses about the way symptoms fluctuate over time when members of the problem-system think or act differently. Tasks may also be assigned to help system members break the cycle of interaction around the symptom.

In Positive Practice, tasks may be classified into seven categories. First, symptom monitoring tasks where clients keep a record of fluctuations in the presenting problem; second, belief exploration tasks where clients are asked to explore the beliefs that underpin the cycle of interaction around the presenting problem; third, exception amplification tasks which involve clients building upon those unique situations where problems should occur but do not; fourth, skills development tasks; fifth, tasks which entail role changes; sixth, rituals that aim to bring about changes in system members' belief systems; and seventh, paradoxical tasks. We will explore each of these types of tasks in detail in this chapter, and then look at some general guidelines for inviting family members to carry out tasks in Positive Practice. But first let us return to the Barrow family and the tasks that they were invited to complete.

The Barrow family were invited to complete three tasks at the end of the first session.

1. Caroline was invited to record a pain rating three times a day on a ten point scale and to note factors that effected the intensity of these ratings.
2. Sheila and Dick were offered the task of discussing the various courses of action that would follow from their different beliefs about the problem and to list the pros and cons associated with each course of action.

3. Mat was invited to withdraw from further involvement in the problem altogether.

The reasons behind inviting the Barrows to complete these specific tasks deserves some elaboration. Principally, I hoped that the outcomes of these tasks would throw light on the degree to which family members were able to cooperate with me in a therapeutic way. Some family members find it easy to accept and complete tasks. Others do not. This needs to be assessed. A useful way to determine this early in the therapeutic process is to invite family members to complete *assessment tasks*.

In Chapter 4, when we were exploring customerhood, it was noted that deShazer (1988) views clients as varying along a continuum in terms of their readiness to commit themselves to therapeutic change. Three key roles may be identified on this continuum: visitors, complainers and customers. One of the cardinal features that distinguishes visitors, complainers and customers is their response to task assignment. Visitors who have been sent to therapy and attend reluctantly will not complete any tasks. Complainers will complete cognitive, but not behavioural, tasks. They are ready to explore ideas about change but are not yet ready to experiment with different patterns of behaviour that might alter the presenting problem. Finally, customers will complete behavioural assignments aimed at problem resolution. The Barrow family's response to the contracts for assessment and further consultation suggested that they were customers, and this hypothesis was born out by their responses to the tasks, all of which they completed.

The specific assignments given in this case are examples of three of the seven classes of intersession that are often used in Positive Practice: symptom monitoring tasks, belief exploration tasks and role change tasks. Let us deal with each of these in turn. A summary of the characteristics of all seven types of tasks is contained in Figure 9.1.

SYMPTOM MONITORING TASKS

Symptom monitoring tasks involve counting the frequency with which symptoms occur, or rating the intensity of symptoms on ten point scales. Symptoms may be monitored by the parents or by the children. Usually moods, feelings, and pain ratings are monitored by the person with the problem, as was the case with Caroline Barrow. Problem behaviours are normally monitored by parents. Giving symptom monitoring tasks is closely related to goal setting, as discussed in Chapter 8. When explicit goals have been set, a symptom monitoring task is frequently given, so that the therapist can keep track of progress towards these goals.

Symptom monitoring tasks often involve more than simply keeping track of the problem or symptom. It is always useful to ask clients to note any factors associated with changes in symptom intensity or frequency. These may include immediate interactions that occur before or after the change in the symptom. Beliefs, memories, expectations and hopes may also be identified by clients as factors that determine the frequency or intensity of symptoms. Physiological factors such as illness, the effects of medication, and so forth may also influence the symptom, so these factors may be worth recording in some cases.

Structured forms help clients to carry out symptom monitoring tasks. Examples of two such forms are contained in Figures 9.2 and 9.3. Typically in Positive Practice,

TYPE OF TASK	CHARACTERISTICS OF TASK
Symptom monitoring	Tracking symptoms and factors that effect their occurrence
Belief exploration	Thinking about the pros and cons of constraining beliefs and solution oriented beliefs
Exception Amplifying	Building upon existing exceptions to the problem
Skill development	Practising new skills necessary for solving the problem
Role change	Changing the amount and quality of time spent together and the family responsibilities held
Ritual	Highlighting dilemmas, mourning losses and celebrating changes
Paradoxical	Compliance-based paradoxical tasks help clients gain control of symptoms Defiance-based paradoxical tasks help clients use their resistance to change in the service of problem resolution

Figure 9.1.   Seven types of therapeutic tasks

therapists devise their own forms to suit the monitoring task devised for each case. Martin Herbert (1987) and Ian Falloon's (Falloon et al, 1993) treatment manuals are a good source for ideas on symptom monitoring tasks and forms.

Monitoring tasks have long been prized by behaviour therapists because they serve an important assessment function (Falloon, 1991). Information from monitoring tasks may be compared to the typical cycle of interaction surrounding the problem in the right hand column of the formulation. This may lead to a refinement of the formulation through the identification of exceptional circumstances or stimulus conditions where symptoms do not occur. This in turn may suggest ways in which the cycle of interaction around the problem may be broken, principally through arranging for the exceptional circumstances or stimulus conditions associated with problem non-occurrence to recur.

In the Barrow case it was hoped that the outcome of Caroline's task would throw light on the typical course of the symptom over a seven day period. In the second session, Caroline reported on her self-monitoring journal. The pain was worse in the morning and improved over the course of the day. It was absent at weekends, on Monday when Dick was around in the morning and on Tuesday when Kirsty called. It was very bad on Wednesday and Thursday when Caroline had fought viciously with Sheila and missed school. Caroline had gone to school on Friday without incident. The self-monitoring task had confirmed the hypothesis about exceptions which emerged in the first part of the intake interview. That is, the problem cycle could be broken when Dick or Kirsty were present. There was also the possibility that on Fridays, when Dick was due home and it was the end of the school week, Caroline and her mother managed to avoid the pattern of interaction that occurred on Wednesdays and Thursdays. This hypothesis was born out later in the interview.

An additional bonus of self-monitoring tasks is that they usually lead to reported improvement and generate hope. In Caroline's case she mentioned that the degree of

1. RATE YOUR FEELING OF_____ON A 10 POINT SCALE

2. MAKE YOUR RATINGS 3 TIMES A DAY: IN THE MORNING, AT MID-DAY AND IN THE EVENING

3. NOTE POSITIVE AND NEGATIVE EVENTS ASSOCIATED WITH LOW and HIGH RATINGS

4. NOTE THE THOUGHTS YOU HAVE ABOUT THESE EVENTS THAT EFFECT YOUR
   RATINGS

DAY	RATING	POSITIVE AND NEGATIVE EVENTS THAT MOST INFLUENCED RATING	THOUGHTS ABOUT THE EVENT THAT MOST INFLUENCED RATING
Mon			
Tues			
Wed			
Thur			
Fri			
Sat			
Sun			

Figure 9.2.   Feelings self-monitoring chart

NOTE EACH TIME _____ OCCURS

WRITE DOWN WHAT HAPPENED BEFORE AND AFTERWARDS

DAY	EVENT	BEFORE	AFTER
Mon			
Tues			
Wed			
Thurs			
Fri			
Sat			
Sun			

Figure 9.3. Parent monitoring form

pain that she was experiencing was now at six on a ten point scale, about two points lower than it had previously been.

Many clients spontaneously self-monitor their symptoms in the time between making their appointment and arriving for the first consultation. Consequently they notice a pretherapy improvement in their presenting problem. deShazer (1988) and other solution focused therapists working within the constructivist tradition, capitalise upon this phenomena by asking clients about the circumstances surrounding the pre-therapy improvement and their conceptualisation of the recovery process which has already begun. In contrast, many behaviour therapists became disenchanted with self-monitoring because of its reactivity (Critchfield, 1989). Working within a positivist framework, they argued that clients' reported improvements were biased accounts tainted by optimism at the prospect of therapy. They were not objective accounts of *real changes* in the presenting problem. This was, in their view, substantiated by showing that neutral observers did not detect the improvements reported by self-monitoring clients. These two different ways of dealing with the same phenomenon epitomise the difference between therapeutic traditions based on constructivism and positivism.

BELIEF EXPLORATION TASKS

The task offered to Sheila and Dick was to discuss the various courses of action that would follow from their different beliefs about the problem and to list the pros and cons associated with each course of action. This is a typical belief exploration task. It offers certain family members a chance to elaborate the belief systems that trap them in the cycle of interaction around the presenting problem, and to do this between sessions. In the second session Sheila and Dick reported that they had talked about the problem at the weekend. Dick said that he had firmly believed that Caroline was avoiding her duty and needed to be sent to school or punished for not going. However, he recognised that this would upset Sheila and make his time at home unpleasant. It would also widen the gap between himself and Caroline. He also said that he had become less certain about his position since the previous session, partially as a result of talking about it with Sheila and thinking about it while at work. Sheila said that she still believed that Caroline had a serious illness, possibly cancer, and that Caroline needed hospitalisation and investigation. However, because Caroline refused to go into hospital, Sheila had begun to have slight doubts about her position. She thought that her approach would be safest, because it would protect Caroline's health. However, it would lead to a major fight between herself and Caroline, and to opposition from Dick.

The Barrows' response to a belief exploration task is fairly typical. As a result of looking at their beliefs about the problem, and the consequences of following through on these, their positions have become less entrenched.

EXCEPTION AMPLIFYING TASKS

In the Barrow case there were clear exceptions to the cycle of interaction surrounding the presenting problem. These included situations where Dick was actually present or likely to be present soon and situations where Caroline's friend, Kirsty, was present. One possible task that could have arisen from information about exceptions would have been to invite the family to arrange for either Kirsty or Dick to be present every day.

This would insure that Caroline was always in an exceptional circumstance and so would no longer experience abdominal pain and need to miss school.

With exception amplification tasks, the therapist first identifies exceptional circumstances where the problem does not occur, and invites the family to recreate these regularly. This type of task is based on stimulus control interventions in behavioural family therapy (Falloon, 1991), deShazer's (1988) exception based tasks and White's (White and Epston, 1990) unique-outcome based strategies described previously in Chapter 5.

SKILL BASED TASKS

Families with children need specific skills and strengths to manage the tasks of family life successfully. These skills include problem-solving, communication, negotiation,

SKILLS	TASK EXAMPLES
Communication Skills * Listening without interruption * Summarising * Acknowledging what has been said * Replying to key points * Using "I" statements * Avoiding blaming or sulking	Take a 10 minute period each evening and tell each other without interruption what you noticed about the children on that day. Each of you may take a five minute turn. Reflect back a summary of what you have heard and check its accuracy
Problem Solving Skills * Defining the problem * Brainstorming options * Exploring pros and cons * Agreeing on a joint action plan * Implementing the plan * Reviewing progress * Revising the original plan	Discuss the pros and cons of the three main options you have identified today. Then agree on a joint plan
Nurturing skills * Making "I need" statements * Avoiding "You must" statements * Meeting needs * Saying "No" * Interpreting infants "need signals" * Balancing give and take	Each of you make list of things that you would like more of from each other. Then make a list of what you would like to give more of to each other
Behaviour Control Skills * Agreeing on clear rules * Setting clear consequences * Following through * Using rewards * Using time-out and little punishment * Talking about self-control * Ensuring safety	Use time out for a week and see if you can find a way to control your own temper. For each time you finish a meal without fighting with you brother, you get a star to put on your star chart

Figure 9.4. Examples of skill based tasks

nurturing and behavioural control. All of these skills are recognised as core dimensions in a number of well developed models of family functioning (Walsh, 1993), notably the McMaster model (Epstein and Bishop, 1981).

In Figure 9.3 some of the skills necessary for communication, problem-solving, and behaviour control are set out, along with a sample task that might be used to assess how well these skills have been developed by family members or to help families change their pattern of interaction around the presenting problem. Throughout the lifecycle, parents need to be able to communicate clearly with each other and to solve parenting problems in a systematic way. In Positive Practice to assess parents' joint problem solving and communication skills, parents are often asked to discuss a number of options, to explore the pros and cons of each, and then to agree on a joint course of action. Where parents succeed in completing the task, sometimes the cycle of interaction around the problem changes and the problem resolves. Where parents have difficulty with the task, the parents' motivation to be involved in therapy may be heightened because they see clearly that they need facilitation in problem-solving and communication. Both behavioural and structural approaches to family therapy place considerable emphasis on the importance of the parents' capacity to communicate clearly with each other and to take a joint approach to problem solving (Falloon, 1991; Colapinto, 1991).

In some families nurturing children is a major problem. Disobedient youngsters, children with difficult temperaments, and infants who cry incessantly or who have sleep problems may all become involved in relationships with their parents where their need for nurturance is not met and this may exacerbate their behavioural problems. With these families, it is vital to check if the children can express their needs and that the parents can hear these requests and respond to them. Thus, assessment tasks may focus on asking children to express their needs and asking parents to listen to these. This task was a central part of Virginia Satir's approach to family therapy (Satir, 1967). Within the Irish culture, where nurturance is often confused with indulgence, many parents that I see in my practice believe that to meet a child's stated need for nurturance will *spoil* the child and will lead to weak character development.

The other side of the coin is where parents are unassertive with children. Tasks that require the parent to recognise their own needs and to say *No* to the child's needs under specific circumstances are useful for assessing flexibility here.

Infants' nurturance needs pose a special problem for some parents. In many cases of physical child abuse that I have seen, the mother was unable to read the child's non-verbal requests for nurturance. These were often misinterpreted as aggression (Cicchetti and Carlson, 1989). A useful task here is to ask the mother to keep track of the number of requests for nurturance that the child makes in a given time slot.

Conduct disorders are the most prevalent childhood disorder and therefore problems of behavioural control are inevitably a major part of the day-to-day work for practitioners working with children and families (Carr, McDonnell and Owen, 1994). In these cases, parents may have problems with agreeing on a set of rules, making these clear to the child, being praise-focused rather than punishment-focused, being very specific in giving praise and following through on stated consequences (Patterson, 1982). Tasks which invite parents to agree on rules, to use reward systems or time- out consistently and to encourage self-control, throw light on the specific skills that parents have had difficulty in developing.

With infants, safety is the central behaviour control issue. In cases of physical child abuse and neglect, setting a task that requires the parent to notice hazards to the infant's safety, and routine ways in which they mange these will give useful information about strengths or difficulties in this area.

With teenagers, behavioural control issues are best managed through negotiation. A common task used to check on negotiation skills is to ask a parent and the teenager to reach agreement on small non-contentious issue, such as what television programme to watch between six and seven on a Wednesday.

ROLE CHANGE TASKS

Role change tasks are central to structural family therapy (Colapinto, 1991; Minuchin, 1974; Minuchin and Fishman, 1981). Here, family members are asked to make changes to their roles as a way of assessing or changing the hypothetical family structure so that it approximates to a healthy ideal. Ideally, according to structural theory, there should be clear boundaries between generations and a clear family hierarchy. Children should not take on parental roles, nor should a parent and child develop a coalition that is stronger than that between both parents. In describing attachment and the emotional aspect of family life, structural theory holds that the family should be neither too enmeshed nor too disengaged. In describing the rules, roles and tasks of family life, structural theory states that the family should also be neither too rigid nor too chaotic. It should be flexible in the way roles are defined and tasks are carried out. For example, from a structural family therapy viewpoint, the task given to Mat Barrow of withdrawing from the problem situation is a way of assessing the degree of systemic enmeshment. In highly enmeshed systems, no one can distance themselves from the family easily. These types of systems are difficult to work with because, often effective problem solving involves simplifying the system by helping some members to disengage.

With role change tasks, family members may be invited to change the amount and quality of time that they spend together and the types of family tasks and responsibilities that they perform. In Positive Practice, the family's responses to these tasks throw light on the extent to which the presenting problem and the cycle of interaction around it may be changed by inviting system members to change their roles. In the Barrow case, I thought that the system would be simplified if Mat withdrew. I suggested that he do this to see if this was possible. The Barrow family turned up for their second appointment without Mat. This was a hopeful sign. When I inquired about this, Dick said that he had taken the advice I gave and decided to keep out of the situation that Caroline was involved in. This suggested that the family could tolerate some degree of increased distance between its members. It also suggested that the system could be simplified by shedding members. Thus, from a structural viewpoint, the Barrow's was not a rigidly enmeshed family.

What follows are some examples of role change tasks from the family therapy literature. In families where one child takes on a great deal of responsibility to compensate for a weak or absent parent, a common role change task is to ask the child to shed this responsibility and to return to the role of a child. Children who end up in the ambiguous situation of being a child with parental responsibilities have been termed *Parental Children* within the structural family therapy literature (Minuchin and

Fishman, 1981). In the Barrow family, Mat was moving towards the position of being a parental child.

Minuchin (1974) frequently invited peripheral fathers to spend special time with problem children who were involved in enmeshed conflictual or anxiety laden relationships with their mothers. Where families were sufficiently flexible to participate in this task, often rapid improvement occurred since it led to a major change in the cycle of interaction around the presenting problem. Indeed, the practice of prescribing designated periods of special-time for peripheral fathers and problem children as a routine assessment task may be the hallmark of a true-blue structural family therapist.

Selvini-Palazzoli et al (1978a) and the original Milan team in their earlier work treated many families where children's problems persisted because each parent held a different view of how the child's difficulties should be managed. These families evolved behaviour patterns where each parent would undermine the other's attempt to resolve the child's difficulty in a symmetrically escalating spiral of interaction. The Milan team developed a highly effective task for helping families escape from this cycle of interaction around the presenting problem. They invited parents with different views of how to manage child focused problems and distinctly different approaches to solving these to take charge of problem children on alternate days. This is known as the odd-days and even-days prescription. It provides a way for parents to break out of interlocking conflict-ridden roles.

In their more recent work, Selvini-Palazzoli et al (1989) have described rigid patterns of family functioning characteristic of families with psychotic members. Selvini-Palazzoli has developed what she describes as an *Invariable Prescription* to disrupt the rigid cycles of interaction in families of individuals with psychotic members. The invariable prescription is a task that requires the parents of teenage psychotic patients to withdraw from the family as a couple on a regular basis, and to maintain secrecy about these periods of withdrawal. The parents are asked to leave a note for the children saying that they have gone on a trip for a half-day or a day and will be back later. Parents are asked not to discuss these trips away with the children or members of the extended family and to keep notes on the impact of this withdrawal on the functioning of the family and the symptoms of the psychotic member. This task, which clearly differentiates the roles of the parents as marital partners from the rest of the family, has (according to Selvini Palazzoli's clinical reports) profound effects on both the pattern of interaction around the psychotic behaviour and the symptoms of the psychotic young adult. Haley (1980) in his book on helping young adults who are stuck at the *Leaving Home* stage of the family lifecycle, also advocates inviting parents to develop a strong coalition. In both Haley's and Selvini-Palazzoli's work, the aim is to provide parents with a way to develop roles where they are closer to each other than to the symptomatic young adult.

RITUALS

Skills based tasks and role change tasks aim to assess or change aspects of the cycle of interaction that surrounds the problem. The focus is on assessing and changing *behaviour*. However, the three column formulation model gives *belief systems* a central place in constraining system members within their roles in the cycle of behaviour around the presenting problem. In Positive Practice families may be invited to carry out rituals to change these belief systems.

Rituals typically centre on acknowledging a dilemma, mourning a loss or celebrating a change. In the Barrow case, the family could have been invited to carry out a ritual to highlight the dilemma of the parents being unable to agree on a shared understanding of the difficulty Caroline faced. The ritual could have involved the family coming together on a Monday morning and reciting: "We cannot help Caroline because we cannot agree what the problem is. Dick says she's disobedient. Sheila says she is sick. Dick says she should go to school and do her duty. Sheila says she should go to hospital and save her health. We cannot help because we cannot agree. If we agree we are disloyal to our own families". Such ritual statements of family dilemmas often empower family members to re-evaluate their deep seated beliefs and premises sufficiently to try a new approach to solving the problem. The original Milan family therapy team were among the first to offer a central place to the use of rituals to make the families' dilemmas explicit (Selvini-Palazzoli et al, 1977).

Loss through death or separation is an inevitable and painful aspect of the family lifecycle. In adjusting to loss, distinct processes or overlapping stages have been described including shock, denial of the loss, futile searching for the lost person, despair and sadness, anger at the lost person and those seen as responsible for the loss, anxiety about other inevitable losses including one's own death and acceptance (Raphael, 1984). These processes, which are central to the grieving process, occur as family members modify their cognitive model of the world and their belief systems so as to accommodate the loss. The grieving process is complete when family members have developed a cognitive model of family life and belief system which contains the lost member as part of family history rather than ongoing family life. Sometimes families become stuck in the mourning process. In some cases families have tried to short circuit the grieving process and act as if they have grieved, but find that from time to time they become inexplicably and inappropriately angry or sad. In other cases, the expression of sadness or anger persists over years and so compromises family development. Prescribing morning rituals where lost members are remembered in detail and family members then bid them farewell may be liberating for families paralysed by unresolved grief. Such rituals may allow family members to alter their belief system and to accept the loss into their cognitive model of the family. This change in the belief system then frees the family to break out of the cycle of interaction that includes the stuck member's grief response and the family's reaction to it. For example, the husband and two daughters of a courageous woman who died of cancer, after two years were repeatedly involved in acrimonious fights and episodes of withdrawal which sometimes lasted for days. As part of therapy, the daughters and the father were invited to visit the mother's grave regularly on a fortnightly basis for three months. Each of them was to recount one reminiscence during these visits. Before therapy ended they were invited to read farewell letters to their mother at the grave and then to burn them. This was the final mourning ritual. Of course this therapy did not erase the pain and grief that goes with the loss of a wife or mother, but it did unblock the grieving process and liberate the girls and their father from the treadmill of fights followed by withdrawal that led to the referral.

Where families have been grappling unsuccessfully with difficult problems for a long time and finally a small break-through occurs, prescribing a ritual to celebrate success may be appropriate. Seligman has shown that repeated failure leads to beliefs that one is helpless, the situation is hopeless and that one will never be effective in solving problems of living (Abramson, Seligman et al, 1978). People with these belief systems tend to be poorer problem-solvers than those with more positive belief systems. Furthermore, people with low self-efficacy and strong helplessness and hopelessness beliefs tend to discount or deny evidence of success, growth and personal strength. Inviting families to celebrate change, growth, and family strengths may be useful in helping to counter these tendencies and in changing the way in which the family views itself from helpless and stuck to strong and evolving (Bandura, 1981). For example, an isolated single parent and her four children who were referred because of escalating family violence were invited to arrange a celebration meal at which each of the members would formally congratulate each other, in an after dinner speech, for avoiding violence for ten consecutive days.

PARADOXICAL TASKS

At one point, the practice of prescribing paradoxical tasks was the hallmark of strategic and systemic models of family therapy (Madanes, 1991; Campbell et al, 1991). Paradoxical tasks may be classified as *compliance* or *defiance* based (Weeks and L'Abate, 1982). Therapists may decide which type to use depending on their assessment of the relationship they have developed with the client. Relationships entail both *cooperative* and *competitive* aspects. If the relationship is a stage characterised predominantly by cooperation, then compliance based tasks are indicated. Defiance based tasks are better suited to those stages of the therapist-client relationship where competition and resistance to change predominate.

With compliance based tasks the therapist expects the family to comply with the paradoxical directive. However, such directives are only apparently paradoxical. They usually entail a rationale which renders them non-paradoxical. For example, I have treated many children who presented with involuntary tics by asking them to practice their tics for twenty minutes per day under parental supervision. On the face of it, this is paradoxical. The child with the tic is asked to continue having a tic. However, the rationale that is given to the child and parents is that this voluntary practice will help the child learn to control the involuntary movement.

Where families are stuck in a dilemma like the Barrows, asking them to engage in the ritual described in the previous section where the mother and father state the beliefs that prevent them from developing a new and workable solution, is a paradoxical task. The parents can not work effectively together, and they are asked to enact ritualistically their inability to work together. However, the rationale for such a task is that it may bring into awareness other ways of looking at the situation.

Defiance based paradoxical tasks are given when the therapist suspects that clients will not carry them out. All clients are cautious about change. Some clients and therapists develop relationships where clients actively resist any attempt by the therapist to influence them to change. In such cases some strategic therapists give clients defiance based paradoxical tasks. The least intrusive of these, and one commonly employed in Positive Practice, is to advise clients to be cautious about change, to make haste slowly and to avoid attempting implementing a new approach to problem resolution until the problem is fully understood. The task is apparently paradoxical insofar as clients come to therapy to change the way they tackle problems and the therapist advises the client not to make any changes. However, the rationale given renders the task non-paradoxical, i.e. that impulsive action may make things worse. The usual effect of this task is to promote rapid change in clients' behaviour.

The most elaborate approach to developing defiance based paradoxical tasks has been developed by Selvini Palazzoli et al (1978b). The cycle of interaction around the problem is described. Possible unconscious beliefs and benign intentions that restrain family members within this cycle are given as the reason for the continuation of the problem and the cycle surrounding it. The family are advised to continue to maintain the pattern to avoid some unacceptable alternative situation until such time as such avoidance becomes unnecessary. For example, with the Barrow family, the following paradoxical task could have been given:

- *Caroline, it seems to me that you are making a major sacrifice for your parents. You worry about your mother's well-being, at an unconscious level, until your nervous system tightens your intestines sufficiently for you to develop abdominal pain. You then use this pain to protect your mother from loneliness. You stay at home, missing out on the fun you could be having with your friends, and help her with housework. You also provide her with a reason to contact your father regularly while he is away at work. My guess is that you will need to continue to have this problem until your mother becomes less lonely and your father no longer needs to spend so much time away from home. A simple solution would be for you, Sheila, to recognise this and insist that your daughter give up her pain, but you cannot. Your guilt for not preventing your mother's death will not let you, nor will it allow you to form new and meaningful friendships. Another solution would be for you, Dick, to spend more time at home comforting Sheila, but you cannot. Your role is to provide for the family and you will not let them down. So it seems that there is no way out here. You must keep on as you have been doing.*

These types of paradoxical messages may be useful where families are stuck in rigid patterns of interaction, and where families have developed strong competitive relationships with therapists. However, they tend to escalate the competitive symmetry of the therapeutic relationship and undermine the possibility of cooperation. For these reasons, such interventions are only used in Positive Practice when more cooperative approaches have failed. These types of paradoxical prescriptions evolved from the Milan teams earlier work with rituals.

GUIDELINES FOR GIVING TASKS AND DIRECTIVES

Family members are invited to complete tasks in Positive Practice to assess the readiness and the capacity of the system for change, and also to help system members break out of the cycle of interaction around the presenting problem. In clinical work, family members often do not follow through on tasks which they are invited to complete. When this occurs there are at least two main possibilities. The first is that the task was inappropriate to the family. By that I mean that the family were either unable or unwilling to carry out the task. The second possibility is that the therapist did not communicate the task to the family accurately and effectively. As a result the task was misunderstood, forgotten, or the seriousness of it was not appreciated. In Positive Practice, therapists can cut down on the number of incomplete tasks due to miscommunication, by following guidelines set out below.

These guidelines are based on clinical experience and the literature on task giving in family therapy (e.g. Haley, 1976). They are also based on a review of the voluminous empirical literature on patients' compliance with medical advice (Carr, 1990c, d). This literature contains useful lessons about the therapist-client relationship based on findings concerning cooperation between physicians and patients.

When inviting family members to carry out tasks it is important to keep in mind the typically low level of adherence to medical regimes. On average patients forget about 50% of the information given to them by their doctors about their illnesses and treatment regimes. About 40% do not cooperate with their doctor's advice. Thus, almost half of the time it is reasonable to expect clients not to cooperate when invited to complete homework assignments. This level of expectation will prevent you from unnecessary self-criticism, client-criticism and other countertransference reactions. Now let us turn to ten guidelines for setting tasks in Positive Practice.

1. Design the task so that it will fulfil your intentions as simply as possible

The design of a task depends upon its function. You need to decide, for example, if you are giving a task principally to *assess* some aspect of the problem or to empower the family to *solve* the problem. If assessment is your intention you may want to design a task to help family members gather observations about the cycle of interaction around the problem or the belief systems that bind clients into this cycle. If therapeutic change is the main function of the task then, you may wish to invite family members to develop skills, alter their roles or amplify some exceptional circumstance to empower them to break out of the cycle of interaction around the presenting problem. Or you may offer an invitation to conduct a ritual or participate in a paradoxical intervention that may lead to changes in the beliefs that perpetuate the problem cycle. Before you design the task, your intention—the function of the task—must be clear.

With the Barrow family, one of our intentions was to assess fluctuations in Caroline's abdominal pain over the course of a week and factors related to these fluctuations. Once the function of the task is clear, you then need to decide how simply this may be achieved. With Caroline, we could have asked her to monitor her pain every fifteen minutes during the first two hours of every day, and to monitor concurrently her feelings towards her mother, father and brother and for the remainder of the time to keep hourly pain ratings. While this would have provided rich data, the complexity of the task might have interfered with Caroline's comprehension and memory for the task. We elected to request three ratings a day because this would furnish adequate information and because the task was simple enough to be remembered and understood.

A second intention which we held in the Barrow case was to assess the flexibility and scope of Dick and Sheila's belief systems about the problem. The simplest way we could think of to assess this through a homework assignment was to ask them to discuss their different beliefs about the nature of Caroline's difficulties and their respective solutions along with the pros and cons of these.

A third intention was to assess the capacity of the system to shed members, so we invited Mat to withdraw. All three tasks were designed as simply as possible and were based on clear and explicit intentions.

2. Offer invitations to carry out tasks clearly in simple language, inviting clients to do specific things

Frame the task in straightforward language. Avoid jargon, technical terms, overly complex sentence structures and unusual words. For example it is far clearer and simpler to ask parents to *check if their son has messed his pants* than to ask them to *monitor his encopresis*. The language you use should fit with your clients' normal language usage without overaccommodating to their language style. So, for example, to pepper your conversation with expletives (if you do not normally do so) when working with a family that uses four-letter words in every sentence and a limited vocabulary is to over-accommodate. It is probably enough to make sure you use short sentences and simple words.

Make your invitations to carry out tasks highly specific. Be clear about who is being invited to do what, when and under what conditions. Here is an example of a vague task invitation:

- *Take some time to think about this whole thing over the next while.*

A specific task invitation is far more precise.

- *Between now and the next session, Mary and Kevin, I'm inviting you to set aside two periods of about an hour to talk about the pros and cons of Danny sleeping with you or remaining in his cot.*

3. Describe tasks briefly and break complex tasks into parts

Where you want to invite a family to carry out a complex series of tasks, the major problem is presenting the tasks in such a way that the family will remember them. Keep the whole invitation to carry out the series of tasks as brief as possible, and divide the series of tasks into no more than three meaningful chunks. Clients memorise information in chunks. In an optimal clinical situation, probably the maximum number of chunks that a client will remember is five. However, never rely on clients to remember a task with five elements. At the end of a session fatigue, anxiety and the novelty of the consultation context will all interfere with the efficiency of clients' memories. When a task has been categorised into chunks, place the chunk that is most important first and then emphasise its importance. because this is the part that will be remembered best.

4. Repeat the task at least twice and check that the clients have understood the task

Repetition helps clients to remember what you are inviting them to do. After the task has been presented, ask clients to repeat back to you what they have understood the tasks to be. This checking process may seem artificial to clients, but it is an important way of avoiding misunderstanding. Incidentally, where you have coached clients in communication and listening skills, they will recognise this as a key skill for clear communication. Here is how we checked that the parents of a food-refusing child understood the task we gave.

- *That's a lot of stuff to invite anyone to do. Just so that I'm sure you've got it straight can you tell me the routine I've suggested for dinner-times at your house?*

5. Give a rationale for the tasks

Clients are more likely to remember and carry out tasks when they understand exactly how the task will help with the assessment or resolution of the problem. Here are some examples of rationales. This rationale was given to a depressed bulimic teenager who was asked to keep thrice daily ratings of her mood on a ten point scale.

- *We will take a look at the record you have kept in the next sessions and it will help us have a clearer picture of how your mood varies from day to day.*

This rationale was given to a ten year old who had a chronic grimacing tic. The task was to practice the tic for a set period each day under his fathers supervision.

- *When you practice your twitches every day for twenty minutes with your dad, you will begin to get control over them. You see at the moment, they just seem to happen to you. But if you make them happen every day, eventually you will develop control over them*

There was a practice within the strategic family therapy tradition to obscure the rationale for the task purposefully (Weeks and L'Abate, 1982). In Positive Practice, the rationale for the task is always stated.

6. Emphasize the importance of the task

Clients who view their problems as serious are more likely to follow therapeutic directives. If clients' assessments of the seriousness of their problems is inaccurate, the therapist can enhance the likelihood of cooperation with therapeutic directives by giving information about prognosis, mortality or vulnerability. Minuchin often gave information about the consequences of untreated anorexia nervosa in a dramatic way to mobilise families into adopting a more adaptive family structure (Minuchin et al, 1978). He would highlight the fact that some anorexics die through starvation. Then he would offer the parents the choice of either allowing their child to die or of completing the task.

7. Write down complex tasks

A written statement of the tasks may be given to the clients at the end of the session, or posted on to them later that day. Keep these letters short. Use simple language and short sentences. An example of such a letter (based on a task invitation described below) is contained in Figure 9.6. The use of letters in family therapy began with the Milan team's (Campbell et al, 1991) pioneering work and has subsequently been taken up by a variety of therapists working within the strategic (Weeks and L'Abate, 1982), psychoeducational (MacFarlane, 1991), and constructionist (White and Epston, 1990) traditions. A fuller account of the use of letters and other written communications in Positive Practice is given in Chapter 12. A major pitfall facing therapists who decide to back up face-to-face interventions with written material is that they may make their letters too complex.

An alternative to giving written statements of complex tasks is to videotape or audiotape the task and give clients this to take home. This approach has been used to good effect in giving cancer patients news about their diagnosis (Hogbin and Fallowfield, 1989).

8. Mention any potentially negative side-effects of the task

With many family problems, things get worse before they get better. For example, when parents are invited to teach their children temper control using time-out as one strategy, inevitably there will be an increase in the frequency and intensity of tantrums. In Positive Practice, the therapist gives the family a health warning about carrying out the time-out task.

In medical practice it has been found that two-sided messages which point out both the benefits and side-effects of treatment lead to greater adherence to medical advice than do one-sided messages (Carr, 1990d). One explanation for this is that the two sided message offers the patient a cognitive framework which can accommodate conflicting information about compliance with medical advice, while allowing the patient to continue to regard the physician as competent. Where only a one-sided message is given, information which contravenes the physicians advice cannot be accommodated without viewing the physician as incompetent.

9. State that the outcome of the task will be discussed at the next session and convey an expectation of co-operation and success

Here are some examples of how the expectation of cooperation and success may be conveyed, and how the family's sense of co-operation may be heightened. Milton Erickson's ideas have informed many of these examples taken from Positive Practice (Lankton et al, 1991).

In this first set of examples, the therapist asks the family to imagine that the tasks have been completed and then to imagine how they will be as a result of the task completion process.

- *It will be interesting to see how this changes our understanding of the problem.*
- *When another client completed this task they found that the most important thing was .ABC&D I wonder will this be the most important thing for you.*

In this second set of examples, the therapist acknowledges that the tasks are challenging and so gives the family options about the timing of the tasks or the variation of the task they choose to accept.

- *If you find that this task is too difficult to do on Thursday, you may want to wait for 24 hours/ a week/until you are sure you are ready....*
- *If you think you cannot do this task, there is another comparable route you may wish to take but my own opinion is that this is the best way to go.*
- *Would you rather do this task or that?*

In this third set of examples, the therapist offers family members a chance to think about obstacles to task completion and how these will be dealt with.

- *Who do you think will have the most difficulty doing the task and who will come in to the next session and say that they had no problem doing it?*
- *Who will be stumped by obstacles and who will find a way around them so that these tasks are completed?*
- *Is there anything you need to ask me now that will help you manage the obstacles you will have to overcome to complete this task?*

10. Always review tasks

Task review is a core part of Positive Practice and will be discussed fully in Chapter 10. Here, however, it is important to mention that clients are more likely to follow through on tasks if they know that the therapist is going to follow through on task review.

Let us now put all ten guidelines, summarized in Figure 9.5, together with the help of a case example. In this case, an invitation to carry out a series of tasks was given to a family where the son was referred because of school failure. It illustrates how a fairly complex series of tasks can be conveyed in simple language, with each part presented as a chunk and a clear rationale given.

The invitation is fairly brief and simple. The directive contains very specific suggestions. Particular family members are invited to do particular things at specific times for specific durations for specific purposes. The three separate elements of the directive are clearly categorised. The important point concerning father-son contact is presented first and emphasised. The core elements are repeated twice. The invitation also conveys an expectation that it will be reviewed and that the family will achieve success in completing the tasks. The letter contained in Figure 9.6 is written to this family.

- *There are three things that we are inviting you to do between now and the next session. First, John and Dad should spend one hour together each evening. This is vital if John is to regain his confidence. Not three hours, not two hours. One hour and one hour only. OK? Second, Mr and Mrs Longfellow, we advise that you visit the school together as a team on Wednesday evening. You have to both go because both of you will need to hear how John's teacher thinks progress can be made! Third, we suggest that you clarify with the school how you can best help John with his homework. Have you any questions about these three suggestions? John and Dad's daily hour, the school visit and the questions for the school. OK, just so I'm sure I've made myself clear, can you run through the task for me, Mr Longfellow.*

GUIDELINES FOR GIVING TASKS

1. Design simple tasks to fulfil your intentions
2. Offer invitations to carry out tasks clearly in simple language, inviting clients to do specific things
3. Describe tasks briefly and break complex tasks into parts
4. Check that the clients have understood the task
5. Give a rationale for the tasks
6. Emphasize the importance of the task
7. Write down complex tasks
8. Mention any potentially negative side-effects of the task
9. State that the outcome of the task will be discussed at the next session and convey an expectation of cooperation and success
10. Always review tasks

Figure 9.5.   Guidelines for giving tasks

Clanwilliam Institute
Clanwilliam Terrace
Dublin 2

The Longfellows
7747 Dublin Road
Sutton
Dublin 13

Dear Tom, Rachel and John:

Just a note to recap the three things we decided at the end of today's session.

• First, John and Tom should spend one hour together each evening. This is vital if John is to regain his confidence.

• Second, Tom and Rachel, we advise that you visit the school together as a team on Wednesday evening. You have to both go because both of you will need to hear how John's teacher thinks progress can be made.

• Third, we suggest that you clarify with the school how you can best help John with his homework.

I look forward to hearing how you get on.

See you on 2.3.93. at 6.pm.

Yours sincerely

Dr Alan Carr

Figure 9.6.   Letter to the Longfellows

SUMMARY

Family members may be assigned tasks between sessions both to *assess* how the problem system functions and to empower clients to *change* the problem system. In Positive Practice tasks may be classified into seven categories. First, symptom monitoring tasks where clients keep a record of fluctuations in the presenting problem; second, belief exploration tasks where clients are asked to explore the beliefs that underpin the cycle of interaction around the presenting problem; third, exception amplification tasks which involve clients building upon those unique situations where problems should occur but do not; fourth, skills development tasks; fifth, tasks which entail role changes; sixth, rituals that aim to bring about changes in system members' belief systems; and seventh, paradoxical tasks.

The probability that clients will understand, remember, and complete tasks is increased if certain guidelines are followed. When inviting clients to complete tasks, design the task so that it is as simple as possible. Offer invitations to carry out specific tasks clearly in simple language. Describe tasks briefly and break complex tasks into parts. Repeat the task at least twice to clients and check that the clients have understood and remembered it. Clients may also be helped to remember tasks by giving them a written account of the task. Give a rationale for each task and emphasise its importance. But also mention any potentially negative side-effects it may entail. Make it clear to clients that the outcome of the task will be discussed at the next session, and convey an expectation of co-operation and success. Finally, always follow through and review tasks in the first part of the following session.

Exercise 9.1.

This exercise is based on the Stuart case, which we first came across in Chapter 4 and around which Exercise 8.1. on goal setting was based. You will remember that Paul Stuart is aged 9 and was referred by the GP who identified encopresis, attainment problems, and disobedience at home as the main problems. A three column formulation of the case is given at the end of Chapter 8.

Work in pairs. Design the following tasks and write them down as you would hope to deliver them to the Stuart family at the end of a session, early in the therapy process.

- A symptom monitoring task that will give information about Paul's encopresis and the conflict that Paul and other family members engage in

- A belief exploration task that will help Mr and Mrs Stuart explore the beliefs that underpin their management of conflict and soiling

- An exception amplification task which will help the Stuarts create exceptional circumstances where the problems are less likely to occur

- A skills development task that will improve the Stuarts management of conflict

- A role change task that will improve the quality of the father-son relationship in the Stuart family

- A ritual task to help the Stuarts acknowledge the loss that Paul experiences when he can no longer perform as well as he wants to at school.

- A compliance based paradoxical task to help Paul develop control over his temper.

- A defiance based paradoxical task to help the family break the cycle of interaction around the problem (set out in the formulation at the end of Chapter 8).

Exercise 9.2.

Work in groups of at least 6 members. Five people take the roles of members of the Stuart family. The remaining person or people take the roles of the therapist and team.

The therapist and team develop a plan for inviting the members of the Stuart family to complete two of the tasks drawn up in Exercise 9.1.

People role-playing family members need to take 10 minutes to talk together as a family and to develop their roles.

Take about 30 minutes to role-play the interview. The therapist must try to follow the guidelines for giving tasks contained in Figure 9. 5.

Derole after the interview.

Take 20 minutes to discuss

1. What the experience was like for family members and
2. Which aspects of the interviewing process were within the therapist's competence which offered the greatest challenge

10

Mid-Therapy Manoeuvres
Relabelling, Reframing and Coaching

In Positive Practice, the bulk of the time in most consultations is devoted either to coaching family members in new skills to help them break the cycle of interaction around the presenting problem, or to the transformation of belief systems that trap them in this cycle. The beginning and end of most sessions are reserved for task review and task setting. In this chapter we will deal with those activities that occupy therapists and families in the heart of most sessions: skills training and transforming belief systems. Let us return to the Barrow case and trace their progress through the second and third consultations. Following this, we will look at some general guidelines for skills training and reframing.

THE BARROW'S SECOND SESSION

Task Review

The session began with a review of the tasks that had been set at the end of the first consultation. It has already been mentioned in Chapter 9 that the parents and Caroline attended the second session and that Mat, following our suggestion, did not join them. Caroline completed the task of monitoring her pain levels and noting factors associated with improvement. Her average pain rating, during the episodes, was five on the ten point scale. Lower ratings occurred when Kirsty accompanied Caroline to school, or on Mondays and Fridays when Dick had been around early in the morning or was due to be around in the evening. Caroline had attended school on seven of the nine school days that occurred between the first and second session. Sheila and Dick completed their task of discussing the pros and cons of their respective beliefs about the best way to solve Caroline's problem. They agreed that there were serious difficulties with both approaches. Dick's disciplinarian approach would lead to opposition from Sheila, and Sheila's medical approach would lead to opposition from Caroline and Dick.

Goal Setting

This task review was followed by goal setting. The elimination of Caroline's pain was Sheila's main goal. Dick set 100% school attendance as his main goal. Caroline said that she wanted to be free from the endless fights with Sheila and for the pain to go away.

I suggested that for Caroline to learn pain management skills and for Sheila and Dick to reach a negotiated joint course of action to take in relation to managing Caroline's difficulties might be useful intermediate goals. The Barrows accepted these without question.

Pain Management Skills Training

The remainder of the session was devoted to helping Caroline develop pain management skills. I showed Caroline some relaxation exercises and then helped her use visualisation skills to manage abdominal discomfort. This training was done in the presence of the parents. Caroline was able, at the end of a thirty minute training period, to use the relaxation and visualisation exercises without much prompting.

For the relaxation exercises, she began with deep diaphragmatic breathing. She inhaled for a count of three, held her breath for a count of three and exhaled for a count of six. For each breath she was shown how to fill the lower half of her lungs with air by trying to push her navel forward as she inhaled. Once she had mastered this breathing exercise, Caroline replaced the mental counting with a visual image of warm yellow light being taken in and spreading through her body as she exhaled. She was then shown how to direct her attention to various muscle groups, tense them slightly and then relax them. She relaxed the muscles in her arms, legs, neck, face and abdomen. With her body completely relaxed she returned to focusing on breathing and visualising the healing light spreading throughout her body. She then practised focusing this visualisation of light on her abdomen. This approach to dealing with pain was based on behavioural and hypnotic pain management programmes (Ioannou, 1991).

I then invited Caroline to practice the exercises alone on a daily basis and to use them to manage the episodes of pain when they recurred. It was also suggested that the exercises might be made more effective if accompanied by a piece of soothing music. Caroline had a portable personal stereo with headphones which she could use to play herself the selected piece of music.

I emphasised to Sheila and Dick that it was important for Caroline to take full responsibility for the management of her pain and to learn to control it independently from their intervention. They appeared to accept this and agreed to refrain from inquiring about her pain or her management of it, except during consultation sessions.

This approach to pain management provided Caroline with skills to lessen the subjective experience of pain through relaxation and visualisation. This is common practice in behavioural paediatrics (Ioannou, 1991). The approach also provided Caroline with a way to block out her perception of anxiety inducing cues which occurred in her interaction with other family members, notably Sheila. Thus it was hoped that these skills would go some way to disrupt the cycle of interaction around the presenting problem.

However, Dick's urge to follow through on some disciplinarian solution, and Sheila's wish to pursue some intensive series of medical investigations remained as factors that might lead them to disrupt Caroline's attempts to use her pain management skills in the way suggested. It was therefore necessary to help Dick and Sheila construct a new understanding of the problem and to negotiate a new set of responsibilities concerning its management. This was identified as a focus for the next session.

Finally, Caroline agreed to keep a record of her daily pain ratings and factors that she saw as being related to them. This provided a way to monitor the effectiveness of the pain management skills. She also agreed to arrange for Kirsty to go to school with her as often as possible. Caroline believed that Kirsty's company would distract her from the pain and enable her to get into school and become involved in her work without becoming disabled.

THE BARROW'S THIRD SESSION

Task Review

Caroline's average rating during episodes of pain was five on a ten point scale. This was the same as the average rating she gave at the previous session. She confirmed, once again, that Dick or Kirsty's actual or potential presence affected the intensity with which she experienced the pain. Also, if she knew Kirsty was going to accompany her to school she found that the pain management skills she had learned in the previous session were far more effective. She had practised these exercises daily, selected a Van Morrison instrumental as her soothing piece of music, and done her best to use the skills to manage the pain in isolation from Sheila or Dick. However, she had been unsuccessful on three occasions. On three out of nine days, she and Sheila had become embroiled in arguments about the pain which culminated in the pain intensifying and in Caroline missing school. Her school attendance rate was therefore 67%, a decrease from the rate of 78% which she had shown for the period before the previous session. On one of the days when Caroline could not go to school, Kirsty had called for her. So it seemed that Kirsty's protective influence was not always effective. It was clear to me at this point that the pain management skills alone would be insufficient to break the cycle of interaction around the presenting problem. The way in which Sheila and Dick behaved within this cycle would also need to alter. This would probably require them to change their beliefs about the nature of the problem and the types of solutions entailed by these beliefs.

Reframing

I asked Sheila to articulate her anxiety about Caroline's health. She did so at length saying that she was worried that Caroline suffered from an undiagnosed illness. This belief had lessened for a time but was now stronger than ever. Even if a thorough physical examination revealed nothing abnormal about Caroline's health, Sheila would remain anxious because the source of Caroline's pain might not be detectable through routine medical investigations. Sheila therefore agreed that a second medical opinion was not what she wanted. She wanted certainty and she knew that this was unobtainable so her anxiety continued to increase.

I asked Dick to outline his position. He said that he felt more strongly than ever that Caroline was playing on Sheila's fear. He was convinced that Caroline needed a firm hand. He was angrier about the problem now than he had ever been. Following these two extreme framings of the problem, I offered a reframing of Caroline's symptom. This was a simplification of the formulation constructed in the first session. First, I reiterated the view that Caroline was vulnerable to abdominal pains because of her history of gastrointestinal problems. Second, I pointed out that stomach pain was exacerbated by anxiety. Third, I suggested that Caroline's pain only intensified when she was anxious. Fourth, I pointed out how Caroline's anxiety level increased when she saw that Sheila was worried, and that the more polarized Sheila and Dick became in their view of the problem as medical or disciplinary, the more anxiety was transmitted to Caroline through Sheila. This reframing was drawn out as a model on the white board (and is reproduced in Figure 10.1).

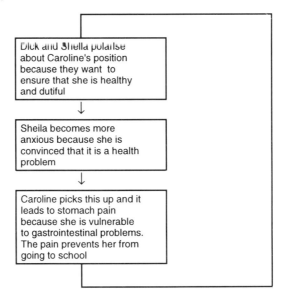

Figure 10.1.   Simplified reframing of the Barrow's problems

I then checked with Sheila, that the more polarised she and Dick became, the more anxiety she felt. She agreed. Caroline agreed that her pain was directly related to the intensity of Sheila's anxiety laden concerned inquiries.

Two possible areas of change were then pinpointed. First, that Caroline manage her pain independently of Sheila in the way that had been suggested in the previous session. Second, that Sheila and Dick negotiate a non-polarised position and agree on how to manage it jointly. This was drawn on the whiteboard and is reproduced in Figure 10.2.

Sheila and Dick agreed to try to work out a joint position on how to manage the problem.

Communication and Listening Skills Training

I asked Sheila to explain to Dick what she would need him to do or say in order for her to be able to allow Caroline to manage her pain independently. She was asked to take her time to collect her thoughts, and then to make her points one at a time as unambiguously as possible. Dick found listening difficult and kept interrupting. So he was coached in how to hear Sheila out. It was explained that the main task in listening was to memorise carefully the key points that Sheila was listing and then when she was finished to summarise these and check if they had been received and understood accurately. After two or three false starts, Dick heard Sheila out without interruption and checked that he had understood her properly. He joked that this was a bit like the

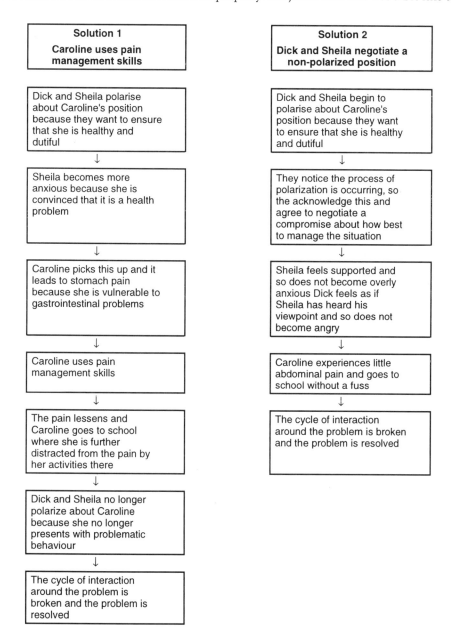

Solution 1	Solution 2
Caroline uses pain management skills	**Dick and Sheila negotiate a non-polarized position**
Dick and Sheila polarise about Caroline's position because they want to ensure that she is healthy and dutiful	Dick and Sheila begin to polarise about Caroline's position because they want to ensure that she is healthy and dutiful
↓	↓
Sheila becomes more anxious because she is convinced that it is a health problem	They notice the process of polarization is occurring, so the acknowledge this and agree to negotiate a compromise about how best to manage the situation
↓	↓
Caroline picks this up and it leads to stomach pain because she is vulnerable to gastrointestinal problems	Sheila feels supported and so does not become overly anxious Dick feels as if Sheila has heard his viewpoint and so does not become angry
↓	↓
Caroline uses pain management skills	Caroline experiences little abdominal pain and goes to school without a fuss
↓	↓
The pain lessens and Caroline goes to school where she is further distracted from the pain by her activities there	The cycle of interaction around the problem is broken and the problem is resolved
↓	
Dick and Sheila no longer polarize about Caroline because she no longer presents with problematic behaviour	
↓	
The cycle of interaction around the problem is broken and the problem is resolved	

Figure 10.2.   Two possible solutions entailed by the simplified reframing of the Barrow's problems

way in which he had been trained to manage customers' objections and concerns in a sales situation when a big order was at stake. However, in listening to Sheila I suggested that he was used to interrupting her and found this a difficult habit to suppress.

Sheila made three central points. First, she wanted Dick to understand just how frightened she was that Caroline was ill. Second, she wanted to be able to contact him on his carphone on those mornings when Caroline was in pain, and talk to him about it. Third, she wanted him to stop criticising her for being concerned for her child's welfare. These points were put up on the whiteboard.

In the second half of the exercise, Sheila listened to Dick while he stated what help he needed in order to be supportive of her. First he said that he needed her to agree that Caroline should go to school regularly, unless the family doctor said she was ill. And second, he wanted her to stop criticising him for saying that Caroline's education was important. These points were arranged on the whiteboard with Sheila's and are reproduced in Figure 10.3.

Sheila's requests	Dick's requests
Dick to understand her intense fear for Caroline's well-being	Sheila to insist that Caroline go to school unless the GP says she is ill
Dick to be available on the carphone in the mornings when Caroline is in pain	Sheila to stop criticising him for valuing Caroline's education
Dick to stop criticising her for being concerned about her child's health	

Figure 10.3.   Sheila and Dick's requests from the communications training exercise

Problem-solving Skills Training

I then said that the points on the board were now the problem, and asked that Sheila and Dick, with Caroline's help, boil the problem down to its bare essentials, list various ways that each of these could be solved, the pro's and con's of each and the best option for solving the problem.

They boiled the problem down to three components. First, that mutual criticism should stop. Second, that Dick make himself available to Sheila by phone while Caroline managed her pain. Third, that in those instances where Caroline could not control the pain sufficiently to go to school, the GP be involved. Numerous solutions to each of these three problems and a variety of pros and cons were generated. They were put up on the whiteboard as they emerged. Some examples are contained in Figure 10.4. After a protracted and humorous conversation an agreement was reached. Criticism of Sheila by Dick or Dick by Sheila for their views concerning Caroline's health and education became a finable offence. The fine was to be fifty pence per criticism. The proceeds were to go to Oxfam. It was also agreed that Dick would call home every morning at 8.30. He was to ask Sheila to express all her concerns about Caroline to him and he would respond with good listening skills and no criticism. Finally, if Caroline had not left the house by 8.35 a.m, Sheila was to take her to the GP's surgery for a checkup. If he gave her a clean bill of health, she was to take her to school herself, and explain to her year-head that she needed a brief period to relax herself before joining the class.

This session ended on a light note, with all three members of the Barrow family expressing confidence that they could follow through on these tasks. Caroline agreed to continue to keep her record of pain ratings. The present session had been scheduled out of office hours so the next session, in keeping with our contract to hold alternate sessions

Problem	Options	Pros and cons
Stop mutual criticism	Try to be more thoughtful	+ It would be romantic - There would be no incentive to be thoughtful when tempers got heated
	Agree a pact	Same pros and cons as first option
	Agree a pact with a cost for every infringement and give money to Caroline	+ There would be an incentive to stick to pact - Caroline might side with Sheila against Dick to encourage criticism to get money
	Agree a pact with a cost for every infringement and give money to charity	+ There would be an incentive to stick to pact + Infringements would be of benefit to charity
Dick and Sheila to make supportive contact	Sheila phone Dick at set time	+ Gives Sheila a sense of control Cost incurred by family -
	Dick phone Sheila	+ More convenient for Dick + Cost covered by company
GP to assess Caroline's health	Sheila to call GP for home visit	+ Very convenient for Caroline who is in pain - Probably would not come till after 11 and so Caroline would miss at least a half day at school
	Sheila to drive Caroline to GP's surgery	+ Fairly convenient for Caroline + Would ensure that Caroline could attend school by 10 am if the GP said it was OK

Figure 10.4. Pros and cons of various optional solutions to three problems identified by Dick and Sheila

within office hours, was set for 2pm a fortnight hence. We agreed that I should contact the GP and the school and explain the plan to them. This was done, without incident, the following morning.

Having reviewed the second and third consultations with the Barrow family, let us now turn our attention to the main interventions that were employed. In particular let us explore structuring the session, reframing the problem and skills training.

STRUCTURING THE SESSION

Once assessment has been completed and a contract for treatment has been established, most of the sessions in the midphase of consultation follow a set structure. The session usually opens with a review of the tasks which the family members were invited to complete. Commonly, this also includes a review of the status of the presenting problem, since one of the tasks is usually to keep a record of symptoms. This opening phase of the session leads into the heart of the session.

Here the therapist, guided by the task review and the three column formulation, helps family members to develop skills to break the cycle of interaction around the presenting problem, or to transform their belief systems so that their beliefs no longer bind them into this repetitive pattern of behaviour. Family members may be helped to develop new skills through coaching. Reframing and certain styles of questioning may be used to help family members evolve new beliefs about their problem situation. In Positive Practice most sessions conclude with the therapist offering the family tasks to complete before the next session. These tasks often build on the skills development or belief change processes that have occurred in the heart of the consultation.

Because mid-therapy consultations are structured into at least three distinct parts, it is useful to follow a three section format in note taking. A note taking template which takes account of this is contained in Figure 10.5.

Some therapists, particularly those that work in a team context, like to take a break between the heart of the session and the final task offering phase. This break is used to develop tasks to offer to the family. The advantages and disadvantages of introducing a break into the session at this point, and the arguments for and against allowing the family to observe team interaction during task development, are similar to those discussed in connection with formulation construction in Chapter 7.

INDIVIDUALISTIC BELIEF SYSTEMS AND KARPMAN'S TRIANGLE

Reframing the problems which families bring for consultation, or relabelling behaviour associated with these problems, are two ways of helping families evolve more useful belief systems about their difficulties. With both of these interventions, alternative positive ways of construing patterns of interaction and individual behaviours are offered. The interventions attempt to capitalize upon our natural tendency, when things are going well, to look on the bright side of life. Incidentally, there is now a vast body of empirical evidence to show that a tendency towards optimism (rather than realism or pessimism) is associated with mental health, relationship satisfaction and productivity at work (Taylor and Brown, 1988). Before looking in detail at how to go about

---

CONSULTATION NUMBER
DATE

ATTENDANCE

The following people attended

The following people were invited but did not attend

Comments

TASKS

The following tasks were completed

The following tasks were not completed

HEART OF THE CONSULTATION

Major themes   Beliefs explored   Skills developed

TASK INVITATIONS

NEXT CONSULTATION
Date
People invited

Figure 10.5.   Template for session notes

relabelling and reframing let us explore some of the more common belief systems that parents who come for consultation hold about their children's problematic behaviour.

Many parents who bring their children to therapy frame the problem as an individual difficulty rather than as an interactional process. Implicit in the accounts given by many parents is the view that their child as intrinsically delinquent, depressed, ill or seriously psychologically disturbed. Put in very simplistic terms, many parents who bring their children for treatment construe them as *bad, sad, sick,* or *mad* (although they may not use such simple or pejorative descriptors). They hold problem-saturated views of their children's identities (White, 1993). When parents construe their children as essentially bad, sad, sick or mad, they are construing them as *victims.* When they view their children as victims, they become constrained into using two destructive relational styles which may be referred to as *rescuing* or *persecuting* (Carr, 1989; Karpman, 1968). If a parent construes a child as being *sad, mad* or *sick,* the typical response is for the parent to attempt to rescue the child by being overprotective or overindulgent. This relational style is destructive because the child is denied the opportunity to take on age-appropriate responsibilities and to exploit opportunities for coping with the stresses and challenges that life offers. If the child is construed as essentially disobedient or *bad,* then the typical response is for the parent to persecute the child through criticism and blame. This leads to the child being denied the experience of acceptance which is important for developing self-esteem.

An interesting feature of these two relational styles is that when a third person becomes involved in an interaction with a victim and either a rescuer or persecutor, they inadvertently take up the empty role in what has been termed Karpman's triangle (Karpman, 1968). Karpman's triangle is set out in Figure 10.6.

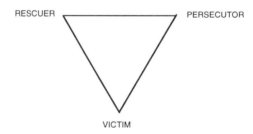

Figure 10.6.   *Karpman's triangle*

For example, in the Barrow family, Dick would inadvertently slip into the role of persecuting Caroline (the victim) when Sheila was in the role of rescuer. This leads to parental polarisation and anxiety on the child's part about taking sides and denying loyalty to one parent. A second interesting feature of the victim-rescuer-persecutor triangle is the tendency of rescuers and persecutors periodically to change roles. For example, from time to time, Sheila would become frustrated through her ineffective attempts to rescue Caroline, and persecute her daughter by nagging or criticising her. This flip-flopping between the roles of rescuer and persecutor on the parent's part is confusing and anxiety provoking for most children.

Of course, parents do not intentionally set out to become stuck in the constricted roles of persecuting and rescuing. This usually occurs when the demands placed upon them by their child's behaviour and other family stresses and work stresses outstrip their capacity to cope adaptively with the situation. In the Barrow case, the travelling associated with Dick's job and the family's bereavement were two such stresses.

When family members are no longer capable of flexible problem solving, or of mobilising social support to buffer the effects of stress, they resort to a variety of unconscious defences to help them defend themselves against the self-image character-ized by failure. What follows are two patterns of defence that often accompany rescuing and persecuting. The analysis is drawn from psychodynamic psychotherapy (Malan, 1979).

When parents adopt a persecuting role, they defend themselves against a self-image characterized by failure by projecting their own anger into the child, defining the child as bad because of its anger and denying the child's positive qualities. When parents adopt a rescuing role, they defend themselves against a self-image characterized by failure by projecting their own sense of helplessness into the child, denying the child's resourcefulness and responding with overprotection. As has been shown, both of these styles of adaptation cannot be sustained indefinitely. Persecuting parents ultimately become remorseful and adopt a rescuing role. Rescuing parents ultimately become frustrated and adopt a persecuting role. Inevitably both parents and children suffer if these styles of adaptation are used indefinitely.

This elaboration of the interactional and intrapsychic features of Karpman's tri-angle is a useful framework to use when considering how best to use interventions like reframing and relabelling which challenge individualistic framings of children's problems.

Reframing

Reframing is an intervention that the therapist uses to co-construct new belief systems with clients, belief systems which will open up new possibilities for dealing with the presenting problem (Weeks and L'Abate, 1982). For example, Dick saw Caroline's behaviour as disobedience. He saw her as *bad*. Sheila, on the other hand saw Caroline as *sick*. These individualistic framings of Caroline's problem were not leading the Barrows towards a useful solution. The reframing contained in Figure 10.1 offers an interactional way of conceptualising Caroline's pain experience and school non-attendance as part of a system which includes her parents' different individualistic definitions of the problem and the behaviour associated with these definitions. This particular reframing is more useful than the individualistic accounts, because it opens up two skills based solutions to the problem. These are set out in Figure 10.2.

Reframing involves three distinct steps. First, listen closely to the clients' current description of the sequence of events and their framing or interpretation of these. Probe and facilitate full elaboration of the viewpoint. Second, separate the behavioural events from the meaning attributed to these by the clients. Third, tentatively offer an alternative more positive way of giving significance to the sequence of behavioural events. Usually this will be consistent with the overall three column formulation constructed during the assessment period. Often it helps the family understand and remember the reframing if it is shown pictorially.

In Positive Practice, assessment and formulation construction is reframing on a grand scale. However, throughout the course of therapy, this process of suggesting new frames of reference through which clients may view events that they have described is a crucial part of the therapists task. A reframing is like a micro-formulation. Often reframings of events that occur between sessions look like one column simplifications of the three column formulation which guides the overall process of consultation. This is illustrated by the reframing of the Barrow's problem in Figure 10.1.

Relabelling

In many families referred for consultation, parents label much of their children's *ambiguous behaviour* as a reflection of them being essentially bad, sad, sick or mad. Relabelling is a process whereby the therapist offers a new label for the ambiguous behaviour: a label which defines the behaviour as unrelated to being bad, sad sick or mad (e.g. Weeks and L'Abate, 1982). For example, in the third session with the Barrows, Sheila, whose problem-saturated construction of Caroline was that of an essentially sick child, said

- *I went into Caroline's bedroom on Tuesday morning and I immediately saw that she was* **poorly**. *She took her time answering me and she didn't sit up.*

As part of the process of co-constructing a more useful way of understanding Caroline's behaviour, I relabelled her disposition at the time as thoughtful. Here is what I said.

- *When you went into her room, Caroline was* **thoughtful** *and took some time to reply to your questions about breakfast.*

Relabelling is an ongoing therapeutic intervention that may be incorporated into your therapeutic conversational style. Relabelling helps families to coconstruct identities for youngsters with difficulties which are not problem-saturated and which do not relegate children to a victim status. The first step is to become sensitised to problem-saturated language (White, 1993). The second step is to identify situations where family members construe ambiguous behaviour as an expression of the problem: that is, as expressions of badness, sadness, sickness or madness. The third step is to offer a relabelling of this ambiguous behaviour as an expression of a normal reaction or a personal strength. If you relabel frequently as part of your therapeutic conversational style, over a number of consultations this may help the family to coconstruct a more useful belief system with you. Here are some more examples of relabelling.

- *He* **hates** *me. He came in and said. "Never again. You're grounded." All I did was stay out a bit late.*

was relabelled as:

- *Your dad was* **worried** *about you when you stayed out a bit late so he said you had to stay in for a week.*
- *He's a little* **brat**. *He had everything out on the floor and was opening all the packets up to annoy me.*

was relabelled as:

- *He was* **curious**, *so he took the stuff out and looked in some of the packets.*
- *She needs to be admitted. She stole £40 and then let herself get caught. I know, something's not right with her.* **She's not herself.**

was relabelled as:

- *She was angry enough to steal and get caught? That's **very angry.***

COACHING FOR SKILLS BASED PROBLEMS

Most clients have an intellectual understanding of the skills necessary for communication, problem-solving, child-management and other aspects of family life, but nevertheless have difficulties using them effectively to solve family problems. The difficulties are of two main sorts. The first set of difficulties involves being unable to identify situations in family life where using these skills is important. For example, in the Barrow case, Dick's training as a sales manager had equipped him with excellent listening skills but he had not realised that it was very important for him to use these in discussing the management of Caroline's difficulties with Sheila. The second set of skills based problems concern the inability to use productive interpersonal skills while experiencing some competing psychological state. Some clients have well developed skills and can identify precisely those situations where they should use the skills but fail to do so because strong emotions such as anger, fear, sadness or elation interfere with their execution of the skills. For example, in the Barrow case, Sheila's fear for Caroline's health and her anger at Dick for not taking her viewpoint, seriously prevented her from solving the problem jointly with Dick. Other factors that interfere with executing skills are fatigue, intoxication, sexual urges, addictive urges or workplace demands. Where couples are tired, drunk, sexually frustrated, craving for drugs or preoccupied with their jobs they find it difficult to use the skills necessary for resolving family difficulties.

In Positive Practice it is important, before coaching family members in the use of various skills, to check their intellectual understanding of them and then to clarify that they know where and when to use them. If they are not aware of where and when to use the skills this becomes an important part of the skills coaching process. For example, in the Barrow case, it was obvious that Sheila and Dick were unable to identify those circumstances where joint planning about helping Caroline were appropriate. So, after the interactional reframing of the problem described in Figure 10.1 was offered, the exact point in this cycle where problem solving and communication skills should be used was pinpointed. This is shown in Figure 10.2.

The easiest way to assess what psychological factors interfere with skill use is to observe families using skills in the consultation. Once the family have been observed using the skills, the therapist gives them accurate feed-back on their performance and asks them to repeat the process. This *do and review* cycle is at the heart of the coaching process and has been developed within the context of behavioural family therapy (Falloon et al, 1993).

The coaching process usually continues after the session through the medium of homework tasks. Task review and the management of resistances associated with clients having difficulty completing tasks that they have accepted will be discussed in Chapter 11. In each of the remaining sections in this chapter we will focus on dealing with resistances to skills usage in the session.

Let us now explore specific approaches to coaching clients in the use of a number of important interpersonal skills.

Communication Skills

The *routine* coaching of clients in communication skills is not a part of Positive Practice. Coaching in these skills only occurs when breaking the cycle of interaction around the presenting problem requires clients to communicate more effectively with each other than they typically do about a specific issue.

Communication skills may be artificially subdivided into those used for telling somebody something and those used for listening. Here are two useful questions to check that clients have an intellectual appreciation of the essential features of both sets of skills.

- *Let me check if we share the same understanding of communication skills? When you want to tell Sheila something really important, first you decide what points you want to make to her. Then you put them in some kind of logical order and mentally rehearse them. Then you tell her what you just rehearsed and check that she has understood you. Does that sort of framework make sense to you?*
- *Let's talk about listening skills. We hear people saying things all the time but when we really want to listen what do we do? Like if I really want to listen to you, I hear you out, without interruption. I summarise the main points that you've made and check that is what you meant. Then, when I'm sure I've received your message accurately, I reply with what I think about it. Can you accept that sort of breakdown of listening skills? Hear the person out. Summarise. Check. Then reply?*

Here is a question that can be asked to find out if clients are prepared to use communication skills at the appropriate times to break the cycle of interaction around the presenting problem, and what they perceive as the main factors that would prevent them from doing so.

- *I'm wondering what you see as the main things that would stop you from using these skills when you see things beginning to go wrong and you know you need to make space to discuss it?*

An important feature of coaching clients in using both communication and problem solving skills is to discuss how they can make time and space for the transactions to occur in an unhurried way. This involves simple things such as removing distractions, turning the television and the radio off, arranging privacy and minimizing interruptions, including phonecalls.

A related issue requiring discussion, is knowing how long an episode of structured communication or problem solving should last. If the episode is too short, no progress will be made. If it is too long, fatigue and negative emotions may occur and destructive transactions may take place. If this happens, any headway that was made may be lost. I usually set ten and fifty minutes as the limits for an episode of structured communication. Fifty minutes is set as the outer limit because this is the maximum duration of most adults' concentration span. I usually invite families to devote brief periods, of about fifteen minutes, to structured communication tasks when they are near the beginning of an episode of treatment. As they move through therapy, longer periods may be more appropriate.

To identify barriers to using communication skills with a particular dyad, ask them to find out what opinions they hold in common and on what points they differ in relation to a topic relevant to the presenting problem. Here is a typical invitation to complete such a task in the therapy session.

- *You both seem to have a good grasp of what it takes to communicate clearly. So I don't fully understand why this does not happen when you sit down to discuss this problem. Show me how you do it. I'm asking you to find out on which three or four points you agree and on which points you disagree when it comes to dealing with Patrick's difficulties. Go ahead.*

Usually this type of invitation is followed by an embarrassed silence. But eventually clients will begin to communicate and after a while demonstrate the mistakes they typically make. These include interrupting before the other person has finished, failing to summarise what the other person said accurately, attributing negative malicious intentions to the other person when they have not communicated that they hold such intentions, failing to check that the message was accurately sent, failing to check that the message has been accurately received, blaming and sulking. In Positive Practice, the therapist lets the episode of communication run for five or ten minutes, and takes notes of various difficulties that occur. Feedback is then given to the family members and, in the light of this, they are asked to complete the episode again. Guidelines for communications training are contained in Figure 10.7.

SPECIFIC GUIDELINES	GENERAL GUIDELINES
LISTENING SKILLS * Listen without interruption * Summarise key points * Check that you have understood accurately * Reply **COMMUNICATION SKILLS** * Decide on specific key points * Organise them logically * Say them clearly * Check you have been understood * Allow space for a reply	* Discuss one problem at a time * Avoid negative mind reading * Avoid blaming, sulking or abusing * Avoid interruptions * Take turns fairly * Be brief * Make congruent "I statements"

Figure 10.7.   Guidelines for coaching in listening and communications skills

Problem Solving Skills

Clients are coached in problem solving skills when it is apparent that they need to take a more systematic approach to resolving some of the difficulties that trap them in the behaviour pattern surrounding the presenting problem. Here is a useful question to check the extent to which clients can appreciate the systematic framework used for problem solving in Positive Practice.

- *Tricky problems need a systematic approach. A lot of people divide up problem solving into steps. First, state the problem specifically. Next, think about lots of different ways to solve it. It doesn't matter if some of these options are strange or unusual. Just get as many options out in the open as possible. Then look at the pros and cons of each and finally select the one that suits everybody best. So that's it. Define the problem, list the options, weigh up the pros and cons and then select the best one. I suppose some of the time you'd do something like this?*

In order to check what prevents clients from using their problem solving skills and to coach them in how to manage these resistances and blockages, some question like the following needs to be asked.

- *OK. So you sometimes use a fairly systematic method for solving problems like dealing with a power cut or cooking Christmas dinner. Now the big question is, what gets in the way of you using these systematic problem solving skills when you try to sort out this problem here?*

When you ask clients to take ten minutes to show you how they use their problem solving skills by addressing some aspect of the presenting problem, many of the blockages and resistances will become apparent. Here is an example of the type of question that may be used to invite clients to do this.

- *One problem you face is finding a way to support each other so you don't get stressed out by this whole thing. Take about ten minutes now to show me how you tackle this problem systematically and come up with a concrete plan that you can both follow through on. A plan that will provide both of you with a sense of being supported.*

When families are observed trying to solve *hot* (emotionally laden) problems often the first pitfall they slide into is that of problem definition. Big vague problems are hard to solve. Little specific problems are easy to solve. Many families need to be coached in how to translate a big vague problem into a few small, specific problems. For example, *to offer regular mutual support* is a big vague problem. This may be subdivided into *(1) Tom spending some time with Mary every day talking about things that bother him, while Mary listens and (2) Mary spending a separate period of time with Tom where she says what is on her mind while he listens.*

A second pitfall where coaching is often required involves trying to solve more than one problem at a time. This amounts to amalgamating a number of small problems into one big problem. It leads to confusion and failure. A third area for coaching is helping families to hold off on evaluating the pros and cons of any one solution until they are sure that they have listed as many as possible. This is important, since premature evaluating can stifle the production of creative solutions. Often families need to be coached out of bad communication habit in problem solving training such as negative mind reading where they attribute negative thoughts or feelings to others, blaming, sulking and abusing others. Where families with chronic problems successfully resolve a difficulty, a vital part of the coaching process is to help them celebrate this victory. Both specific and general guidelines for problem-solving are presented in Figure 10.8.

Behavioural Control Skills

Clients' intellectual understanding of the skills necessary to teach children self-control may be checked with the following type of question.

- *Lets just think about how we go about teaching children to control their tempers or how to follow rules. Everybody has strong opinions about this so I'll just talk about what scientists have found out about it when they have talked to thousands of families in different countries and followed them up over a number of years. Children learn self-control best when the rules about what they can and can't do are clear, when its clear what will happen to them if they do or don't follow the rules, when parents always follow through and reward good behaviour but don't reward*

SPECIFIC GUIDELINES	GENERAL GUIDELINES
* Define the problem * Brainstorm options * Explore pros and cons * Agree on a joint action plan * Implement the plan * Review progress * Revise the original plan	* Divide one big problem into a few small problems * Tackle problems one at a time * Avoid vague problem definitions * Define problems briefly * Show that the problem makes you feel bad * Acknowledge your share of the responsibility in causing the problem * Do not explore pros and cons until you have finished brainstorming * Celebrate success

Figure 10.8.   Guidelines for coaching in problem solving skills

bad behaviour and when improvements in self-control over time are talked about regularly. Does that fit with what you have seen with your own children?

The following question throws light on factors that block parents attempts to help their children internalise rules and develop a sense of self-control.

• *When Tony has a tantrum or breaks his sister's toys you say you sometimes scream at him or spank him and other times you ignore him and occasionally you try to reason with him. Do you think that if you made a plan to do the same sort of thing each time -say like putting him in his room until he controls his temper- that you would be able to follow through...(after answer).....What would prevent you from following through?*

Many parents who have, in their opinion, *tried everything* and failed to teach their children self-control, feel powerless and have lost faith in any method for helping their youngsters control their tempers and other impulses. They usually express this sense of personal helplessness by blaming the child or the method. So, they say their child would not respond because he is intrinsically bad or because the method is useless. Other parents will admit that they would be unable to contain their own anger and frustration and would give vent to this by screaming or hitting. A vital part of dealing with these resistances in Positive Practice is empathizing with the parents' sense of exasperation and defeat without agreeing that behavioural control programmes are ineffective. Here is an example of how this was put to one parent.

• *It sounds like you've tried everything and got nowhere. You feel like he will never learn how to control his temper. You doubt that anything will work. I know that the programme we use here works. It takes time. It takes energy. Your boy will really test you out for a while when you try this programme so things will get worse before they get better. But in the end it works. However, you need to be ready. You need to have got your energy up and to be determined to help him avoid becoming a delinquent. I could understand it if you said you wanted to wait a while.*

Once parents and children agree to become involved in a behavioural control programme, the heart of the coaching process is facilitating planning. Both parents must accept the plan and with teenage children particularly, youngsters need to play an active role in contributing to the plan to help them learn self-control. Here are some useful questions to ask when facilitating planning a behavioural control programme:

- *It sounds like Carmen has a number of urges that she needs to learn how to control. One is the urge to hit people, another is the urge to break things, another is the urge to stay out past bedtime. Now, of all these urges, what is the main one you want her to learn to control?*
- *Some families like to use a chart like this (the chart in Figure 10.9) and every time the youngster makes it through a period without losing control of his temper he gets a point. At the end of the week the points can be cashed in for a prize. Other families prefer to use a token jar. Every time an hour goes by and the youngster has controlled his temper for the hour a token goes into the jar. These can be used to get a prize at the end of the week. Which system do you think would suit your situation?*
- *This is the way time out works. You give two warnings first. Like this, Carmen, please try to control your temper. This is your first warning. Carmen, please try to control your temper. This is your second warning. Then if Carmen can't control her temper, walk her to time out (her*

For each 30 minute period put either an X in the box if _____ showed self-control or put the number of minutes spent in time-out in the box							
	Mon	Tues	Wed	Thur	Fri	Sat	Sun
8.00							
8.30							
9.00							
9.30							
10.00							
10.30							
11.00							
11.30							
12.00							
12.30							
1.00							
1.30							
2.00							
2.30							
3.00							
3.30							
4.00							
4.30							
5.00							
5.30							
6.00							
6.30							
7.00							
7.30							
8.00							
8.30							
9.00							
9.30							
Total							

Figure 10.9.   Chart for monitoring self-control of aggressive and destructive urges

bedroom) like this. No fuss. No shouting. Just walking. Then say: take five minutes to control your temper and when you are done we will play a game of snakes and ladders (or whatever game Carmen and yourself like). If you open the door at five minutes and she shouts at you, close it for thirty seconds, then open it again if she has stopped. Keep this up until Carmen can show self-control for thirty seconds. Then ask her to come out to play with you. Carmen only gets out of time out when she has shown that she can control her temper for thirty seconds after the first five minute period. Can you run through this time out routine so I'm sure I've said it clearly?

- *Carmen, when you go into time-out your job is to control Angry Alice (the name we gave Carmen's temper) so she doesn't keep stopping you from having fun and being friends with your mum and brother. There are different things you could do. You could let Angry Alice scream and scream for five minutes. You could let Angry Alice hit the mattress one hundred times with the pillow. You could tell Angry Alice your favourite story or sing her a song. Now which of these things would you most like to do to teach Angry Alice how to control herself?*

Guidelines for developing a behavioural control programme are set out in Figure 10.10. For a full account of behavioural programmes consult Martin Herbert's (1987) practice manual. Running a behavioural control programme for the first two weeks is very stressful for most families. The normal pattern is for the time-out period to increase in length gradually and then eventually to begin to diminish. During this escalation period when the child is testing out the parents resolve and having a last binge of self-indulgence before learning self-control, it is important to help families maintain the unconditionally supportive aspect of family life. There are two important interventions that may be useful here. First, spouses may be invited to set aside special time where the focus is on mutual marital support. Second, parents may plan episodes of special time with the children. The important feature of spouse support is that the couple set aside time to spend together without the children to talk to each other about issues unrelated to the children. In single parent families parents may be helped to explore ways for obtaining support from their network of friends and members of the extended family.

Facilitating special-time programmes for families where parents and children have become embroiled in chronic battles is an important part of Positive Practice, and is dealt with in the following section.

Nurturing Skills

Guidelines for developing a nurturing skills programme where parents and children spend *special time* together is set out in Figure 10.11. When children spend special time with their parents they should feel like they are being given unconditional acceptance, warmth and friendship. Parents can help children have that experience by setting aside special time, allowing the child a high degree of control over what happens during this time, taking care to avoid or defuse conflict, and promoting laughter warmth and humour. Here is one way of introducing the idea of special time to families.

- *You have been involved in a struggle together for a long time now and maybe you need some practice at being friends? Here is one thing you can do if you like. Both of you set aside an hour every Saturday morning. No more. No less. Just an hour. Then John, you decide what you would like to do with your dad for that hour. Maybe read a story. Maybe play pool. Maybe visit the park. I don't know. But it has to be something you want to do. Your side of this, Paul, is*

SPECIFIC GUIDELINES	GENERAL GUIDELINES
BEHAVIOUR CONTROL PROGRAMME * Agree on clear rules * Set clear consequences * Follow through * Reward good behaviour * Use time-out or loss of privileges for rule breaking * Monitor change visibly **TIME- OUT** * Give two warnings * Bring the child to time-out without negative emotion * After five minutes engage the child in a positive activity and praise him for temper control * If rule-breaking continues, return child to time-out until thirty seconds of quietness occurs * Engage in positive activity with child and praise for temper control	* Build in episodes of unconditional special time into behavioural control programme * Frame the programme as learning self-control * Involve the child in filling in, designing and using the monitoring chart or system * Monitor increases in positive behaviour as well as decreases in negative behaviour * Do not hold grudges after episodes of negative behaviour * Avoid negative mind reading * Avoid blaming, sulking or abusing * Ask for spouse support when you feel bad about the programme * Celebrate success

Figure 10.10.   Guidelines for behaviour-control programmes

to try to do things that make the time fun and special. Like allow John to be in control of what you do, and try to avoid getting into arguments. The only kind of fighting that's fun for fathers and sons is rough and tumble. Maybe you might do some of that. I don't know. But the thing is, your part is to make John feel like you both can still be friends, despite the bad stuff that we have talked about today.

There is a myth in parts of our society that treating children with respect—honestly telling your children that you love them or that you like things that they do and giving them control over interactions with adults—will *spoil* them. The degree to which families accept this myth and are committed to it needs to be explored, if you are suggesting a special time task. Here is a question that may be used to explore this issue.

- *Some parents get worried that special time will give their children the idea that somehow they have got away with breaking the rules and that it will spoil them. That is, they think it will undo all the good that the self-control training has achieved. To what extent do you think this might happen with John?*

If parents are committed to the belief that special time spoils children, then helping parents accept special time tasks may take considerable negotiation. Episodes of special time are unique opportunities for parents to use empathy as a way to rebuild a sense of trust and understanding rapidly in their relationships with their children. One of the easiest ways for parents to convey that they empathise with their children is to run a commentary on their child's activities and to summarise and expand what their children

SPECIFIC GUIDELINES	GENERAL GUIDELINES
* Set a specific time * Help your child decide what he or she wants to do * Summarise options and pros and cons of these * Agree on an activity * Participate wholeheartedly * Run a commentary on what the child is doing or saying * Make congruent "I like it when you" statements * Laugh and make physical contact through hugs or rough and tumble * Finish the episode by summarising what you did together and how much you enjoyed it	* Try to use the episode to give your child the message that they are in control of what happens and that you like being with them * Try to foresee rule-breaking and prevent it from happening * Notice how much you enjoy being with your child

Figure 10.11.   Guidelines for coaching in nurturing or special time skills

say to them. Parents may be coached in how to do this in a consultation at the end of which special time is offered as a homework task. This form of empathy training can be suggested in the following way.

* *I know you want to improve the sense of understanding between yourself and your son. If he knows you understand him, there will be fewer fights. You can show him you understand him during special time in two very special ways. They sound silly at first, but most children say these ways of talking make them feel understood. Here's the first one. Really watch Paul when he's playing and run a commentary on it. Like, if he's building with lego you might say: "Looks like your putting the two long bits on the bottom and then some wheels. That will make a good car. I wonder what you're going to use for a roof? Oh yes I see. A flat green piece." Have you got the idea? Run a commentary, like a TV commentator. The other thing you can do is summarise and expand. So if John says "Its a truck that picks up the rubbish in the morning." You might say "Its a garbage truck. A big noisy garbage truck that wakes everybody up!!". The 'garbage truck' bit is a summary. The rest is an expansion of the idea. Let's practice that now....*

SUMMARY

Once a contract for therapy has been established and therapeutic goals have been set in the light of a three column formulation, there are a number of interventions that may be used to help families reach their goals. Reframing and relabelling are interventions that aim to change family members' belief systems that trap them in the pattern of interaction around the presenting problem. Reframing involves taking a sequence of behaviour and stripping it of the meaning given to it by the client. The sequence is then re-presented but with a new meaning and from within a new frame of reference. Relabelling is the process where the therapist takes ambiguous behaviours that have been interpreted by clients negatively and redescribes them in positive ways.

Karpman's victim-rescuer-persecutor triangle is a useful framework to keep in mind when reframing and relabelling. Often, referred children are assigned to the victim role of this triangle by their parents who may construe them as bad, sad, sick or mad and frame or label their behaviour in these problem-saturated ways.

The cycle of interaction around the presenting problem may be directly altered by coaching clients in using a variety of interpersonal skills. These include the skills required for accurate communication, effective problem-solving, behavioural control and nurturing children. Coaching involves clarifying clients' intellectual understanding of these skills, observing them using the skills, giving corrective feedback and facilitating further practice.

Some clients follow through and practice skills between sessions. Others do not, even though they are committed to achieving therapeutic goals. Within the field of psychotherapy, the non-completion of therapeutic tasks has been termed *resistance* (Anderson and Stewart, 1983). Methods for managing resistance will be the focus for Chapter 11.

Exercise 10.1. Reframing

Work in pairs and take the roles of therapist and client.

The client must think of a person in their family or at work with whom they have some difficulty and write down one pejorative adjective to describe them (e.g. bossy, boring or a nuisance).

The therapist must then interview the client so as to establish the pattern of interaction that the client observes that leads him or her to use the pejorative adjective to describe the person. Finally, the therapist must reframe the individualistic description of the person in positive and interactional terms.

Exercise 10.2. Relabelling

Work in pairs.

Each person draw up a list of sentences in which a person's ambiguous behaviour is described in negative terms.

Take turns reading out one sentence at a time to your partner who must relabel the ambiguous behaviour in positive terms.

For example, *When he tells me what to do he is bossy* may be relabelled as *When he tells you what to do he is concerned and wants you to get it right first time.*

Exercises 10.3-10.6.

The following four exercises are based on the Stuart case, which we first came across in Chapter 4 and around which the exercises in Chapters 8 and 9 were based. You will remember that Paul Stuart is aged 9 and was referred by the GP who identified encopresis, attainment problems and disobedience at home as the main problems. A three column formulation of the case is given at the end of Chapter 8.

Work in groups of at least 6 members. Five people take the roles of members of the Stuart family. The remaining person or people take the roles of the therapist and team.

For each exercise people role-playing family members need to take 10 minutes to talk together as a family and develop their roles.

For each exercise take about 10 minutes to role-play the interview.

Derole after the interview.

Take 20 minutes to discuss

1.   What the experience was like for family members
2.   Which aspects of the interviewing process were within the therapist's competence and
        which offered the greatest challenge.

Exercise 10.3. Communication skills

Coach the mother and son in communication skills around a neutral non-emotional issue.

Exercise 10.4. Problem solving skills

Coach the whole family in problem-solving skills around a neutral issue.

Exercise 10.5. Behaviour control skills

Coach the parents and son in behavioural control skills.

Exercise 10.6. Nurturing skills

Coach the father and son in nurturing skills.

11

Managing Resistance

In Chapter 10 we traced the progress of the Barrow case through their second and third consultations. Skills training and reframing were the main interventions illustrated by the work which took place in these sessions. The third session concluded with the family agreeing to complete three tasks and with a commitment on my part to contact the school and the GP to explain how their help might be required in completing one of the tasks.

Both the GP and Caroline's year-head were pleased to receive my calls when we finally made contact. However, as is commonly the case, this was a difficult process involving about ten phonecalls. On numerous occasions either the GP and year-head were unavailable or I was committed elsewhere. In Positive Practice, follow-through is crucial even if it takes fifty calls, because families will find it difficult to follow through and complete tasks offered to them if the therapist agrees to take on responsibilities and then does not follow through.

The GP agreed to give Caroline a routine checkup if she had abdominal pain, but said that he knew Caroline well and believed her to be essentially healthy. He was very critical of Mrs Barrow whom he described as overbearing and overprotective. I suggested that the circumstances surrounding her bereavement and the stillbirth might account for this level of concern, and he said that he had not previously taken those factors into account. To some degree this softened his critical attitude towards Sheila. The year-head said that Caroline would be fine if she did not keep trying to dodge work by feigning illness to get time off school. I explained Sheila's concern about Caroline's health and the plan to involve the GP in assessing Caroline's health should she become symptomatic. This led to a softening of the year-head's critical attitude to Caroline.

FOURTH SESSION WITH THE BARROWS

Task Review

Sheila and Caroline attended this Thursday afternoon session which occurred a fortnight following the previous consultation. Sheila said that Dick was unable to attend because of his work commitments. Before exploring the changes in Caroline's symptoms, and the way in which the Barrows handled these, the tasks they were offered in the previous session were reviewed.

Caroline had kept a detailed record of school attendance and fluctuations in the level of pain that she had experienced since the previous session. Her average pain rating for all episodes that occurred in the preceding two weeks was six, an increase of one point compared to those ratings reported in the two previous consultations. Caroline had attended school on six out of ten days. This represented a 60% attendance rate and a deterioration from the attendance rates of 67% that was reported in the third session and 78% that was reported in the second session.

Sheila and Dick had made a criticism money box, and had used it for about three days. About two pounds was in the box. However, enthusiasm for both mutual criticism and for continuing the task had waned. This task had therefore been useful in reducing the criticism which contributed to the parents' polarisation.

Dick had phoned Sheila on Friday, Tuesday and Wednesday, but then he stopped making the regular morning calls to Sheila. Sheila had asked Dick to make morning calls because they gave her a sense of being supported, but he said that it was not practical. This task was apparently successful in fulfilling the function of offering Sheila support, but was either poorly designed or not offered to Dick in a way that allowed him to follow it through.

On only one of the four occasions where Caroline's pain led to school non-attendance was the GP involved. On Thursday of the previous week, Caroline had felt strong pain (about nine on the ten point scale). Sheila brought her to the GP who said she was in no medical danger and could go to school, but should take it easy. Sheila took her home instead. On the three other days that Caroline did not attend school, Sheila and Caroline did not go to the GP's surgery.

Questioning Resistance

This review showed that, from a symptomatic viewpoint, little progress was being made. It also showed that Caroline, Dick and Sheila had difficulty following thorough on some of the tasks that they had agreed to complete. The heart of this session focused on questioning Caroline and Sheila about the beliefs that prevented them and Dick from following through on a course of action which they accepted as a stepping stone towards the resolution of the presenting problem.

There is always the danger that aggressive countertransference reactions to incomplete homework will compromise the therapist's neutrality and therapeutic curiosity (Selvini-Palazzoli et al, 1980a; Cecchin, 1987). If this happens the therapist may become involved in the cycle of interaction around the presenting problem in a way that contributes to its maintenance. If the therapist questions family members in a way that makes them feel blamed, then they may respond by blaming the therapist for not helping them. They may alternatively respond by saying that they believe themselves to be powerless to do anything. A third common response is to distract the therapeutic focus away from the failure to follow through on agreed tasks. The issues of both resistance and countertransference are discussed in some detail below.

Caroline and Sheila were asked to speculate on what prevented Dick from following through on making contact each morning with Sheila by phone. Both Caroline and Sheila thought that Dick desperately wanted promotion so that he would not have to travel so much. In order to get this promotion he was reluctant to take time off to call Sheila because it may have interfered with his work schedule. I asked what beliefs he might have acquired from his parents that also prevented him from phoning Sheila to offer support. Sheila said that she believed that in Dick's family, talking or negotiating about a problem was seen as a sign of weakness. He may not have phoned because he might not have wanted to appear weak. When I asked what might lie behind Dick's family's belief that talking about a problem in detail or a supportive way is a sign of weakness, Caroline said that she thought that her father, and indeed most adults, believed that there was only one right answer to any problem. This process of questioning the layers of beliefs that may underpin resistance is discussed in more detail below.

I then asked Caroline and Sheila to speculate on possible ways that Dick could offer support to Sheila without compromising his work performance and promotion prospects, without appearing weak and without feeling like offering support to Sheila meant that he was in the wrong. Various options were suggested. These included Sheila calling Dick very early in the morning every morning before Dick started work stating her concerns and requesting advice; Sheila agreeing not to call Dick unless she and Caroline were fighting and then asking Dick to act simply as a sounding board; and Dick taking a week's leave and taking on full responsibility for helping Caroline get to school and manage her pain, while Sheila stayed out of the interaction altogether.

Because Dick had not attended the session, I said that I would write to him asking his opinion on which of these options would suit him best, or if there was some alternative that he saw which was more feasible. The letter to Dick which was sent immediately following this session is presented in Figure 11.1. In Chapter 12 we will address the use of letters in Positive Practice for a variety of purposes.

Following the exploration of ways around the resistances that were blocking Dick, we turned our attention to factors that prevented Caroline and Sheila from following through on the plan to visit the GP, Dr Wilson, and enlisting the help of the year-head, Ms Hackett. First I asked for a blow by blow account of the morning where they were successful in visiting the GP, and followed this up with questions about the difference between this morning and the three others where the GP was not visited. There were three main differences. The first was that Sheila and Dick did not make telephone contact. The second was the severity of Caroline's pain. It was much worse on the three mornings she did not go to school. The final difference between the two sets of occasions was the intensity of the conflict between Caroline and Sheila. On the mornings Caroline did not go to school, herself and Sheila became embroiled in intensely conflictual interactions.

One of the reasons why Caroline fought so intensely with Sheila was that she hated the visit to the GP. He gave her a routine checkup and then said that the pain was all in her mind. She could not accept this since she experienced it as *real*. She felt

---

```
                                              Child and Family Clinic
                                              Market Town
                                              Norfolk
                                              22.3.90
Dear Dick

I may have asked you to overcommit yourself by suggesting that you attend every consultation. If
this is the case can you please let me know how many of the remaining three sessions you will be
able to attend. This will help me to plan the most effective use of  each consultation.

I gather from talking to  Sheila and Caroline  that you are particularly busy at work at the moment
and this has prevented you from being able to phone Sheila regularly each morning at 8.30. I am
sorry that we did not take your increased workload into account when we made this plan.

However, Sheila's need for support in managing Caroline remains.  The question is: how can this be
offered in a way that fits with the demands of your work situation. Some suggestions were made in
today's consultation. These included

•      Sheila calling you every morning before you have started work to state her concerns and ask
       for your advice
•      Sheila agreeing not to call you unless she and Caroline are having difficulties and then asking
       you to act as a sounding board for her
•      You taking a weeks leave and taking on responsibility for helping Caroline get to school and
       manage her pain, while Sheila stays out of the interaction altogether.

You may wish to think about these options and consider others you may have in mind with a view to
coming up with one that is feasible.

The next consultation is scheduled for Friday April 6th at 6.00pm. I look forward to seeing you then.


Dr Alan Carr
```

Figure 11.1.   The letter sent to Dick following the session he did not attend

humiliated. The meeting with the year-head, Ms Hackett, went well. She was given a
quiet place to rest until she felt well enough to go to class. The pain had eased off quite
quickly once she had some time on her own to practice her pain management skills.

I asked Caroline how she would like to arrange things on the mornings when she had
severe pain. She said she would like to stay home and do schoolwork there. But if she
had to go to school, she did not want the GP involved. Sheila objected to this, and said
that she might end up with a burst appendix or some other serious condition and she
could not be responsible for that.

Framing a Dilemma

I pointed out the dilemma faced by the Barrows. On the one hand they said that they
would like Caroline to overcome her pain and attend school regularly. They accepted
that the pain intensified when Caroline saw that her mother was very concerned for her
health, probably because this made Caroline concerned for her mother's well-being.
They also accepted that Sheila only became very anxious about Caroline when Dick was
unavailable to support her, or when he polarised with her about the nature of the
problem and how to deal with it.

The other side of the dilemma which I spelled out was that finding a way for Dick to be involved to support Sheila was difficult. His work, essential for the financial viability of the family, obstructed him. There were also difficulties in arranging for the GP to indicate regularly to Sheila whether Caroline's pain was due to a life threatening medical condition or not. Caroline thought that the GP believed she was either faking or mentally deranged. Because of this she felt humiliated and would not see him again.

Finally, I said that this dilemma brought the process of resolving the problem to a standstill for the time being. Some way out of this dilemma needed to be found. This way out might involve a range of courses of action including the following: Sheila and Dick negotiating a jointly acceptable solution; Dick taking a more active role; Caroline and the GP changing their relationship; or Sheila placing more faith in an anxiety based explanation for the pain. I said that I was unsure as to how the dilemma would be resolved and looked forward to discussing this with themselves and Dick in a fortnight.

In the meantime I suggested that Sheila put aside two thirty minute periods to discuss the dilemma with Dick before the next appointment. I also suggested that Caroline continue to monitor her pain level and keep a record of her school attendance.

QUESTIONING RESISTANCE AND FRAMING A THERAPEUTIC DILEMMA

One of the extraordinary paradoxes of all forms of psychotherapy is that clients come to therapy requesting help with their problems, but often when help is offered clients will not cooperate. This apparently paradoxical process has traditionally been referred to as resistance (Anderson and Stewart, 1983). I say *apparently* paradoxical, because in any therapy case, once the clients' resistance is fully understood, it usually makes a great deal of sense and does not appear paradoxical at all.

Clients show resistance in a wide variety of ways. In family consultations it may take the form of not completing tasks between sessions, not attending sessions, or refusing to terminate the therapy process. It may also involve not co-operating during therapy sessions.

For clients to make progress with the resolution of their difficulties the therapist must have some systematic way of dealing with resistance. In Positive Practice the following step-by-step process is used. First, describe the discrepancy between what clients agreed to do and what they actually did. Second, ask about the difference between situations where they managed to follow through on an agreed course of action and those where they did not. Third, ask *what they believed blocked them* from making progress. Fourth, ask if they believe that there are ways that these blocks can be overcome. Fifth, ask about strategies for getting around the blocks. Sixth, ask about the pros and cons of these courses of action. Seventh, *frame a therapeutic dilemma which outlines the costs of maintaining the status quo and the costs of circumventing the blocks.*

This systematic process for questioning resistance is only helpful if the therapist adopts a position characterised by neutrality and curiosity (Selvini et al, 1980; Cecchin, 1993). If clients feel that they are being blamed for not making progress, then they will usually respond by pleading helplessness; blaming the therapist or someone else for the resistance, or distracting the focus of therapy away from the problem of resistance into less painful areas. These three types of further resistance often elicit countertransference reactions on the therapist's part which compound rather than resolve the therapeutic impasse. Let us now look in some detail at specific inquiries used to question resistance, and follow this with a discussion of escalating resistance and countertransference.

INQUIRIES ABOUT RESISTANCE

When clients agree to follow a course of action that will lead to problem resolution and then do not follow through on this, begin the process of questioning resistance by stating your curiosity about this paradox. Here are some examples of how this is done.

- *I know that you all want to solve this thing. So I'm curious about what sorts of things happened to create a situation where you were prevented from doing the task you said you wanted to do?*
- *I want to understand what was happening here. You said at the last meeting that you wanted to help Charles learn how to be honest. We agreed that it would be useful for you to check with his teacher on three occasions about what homework he had, so that you could check if he was being truthful with you about this. But there was some difficulty in this being carried out. It only happened once. I wonder what went on?*

Where clients cooperate on some occasions but not on others the second step is to ask what was the difference between situations where cooperation did and did not occur. Here are some typical questions about this issue.

- *When you look at those situations where your husband and son were able to get together for special time and those where they were not, what was the main difference between them?*
- *What made it easy for you to talk to Charles' teacher on Tuesday but difficult on the other days?*

The third set of inquiries used to question resistance focus directly on the client's beliefs about factors that prevented them from following through on agreed actions. Clients are usually prevented from following through on tasks or making therapeutic progress because of some combination of five types of factors: unpredictable events, lack of ability, lack of commitment, specific beliefs relevant to the problem and emotional pain. Each of these factors will be dealt with in detail in the next section. Useful preliminary inquiries to begin to narrow down the main factors underpinning resistance include the following:

- *What sort of things prevented you from doing this thing that you wanted to do?*
- *My guess is that something stopped you doing it. What things do you think stopped the family meeting together on Thursday night?*
- *Sometimes its difficult to follow through on a plan because something unpredictable happens. Did anything like that happen last week?*
- *Do you think that X had the skill to do Y?*
- *Who do you think is the person who most wants this situation changed?*
- *What belief that X holds do you think prevented him from doing Y?*
- *Sometimes people don't do things because they are worried something bad will happen. I wonder what you think your partner was frightened would happen ?*

Once clients' beliefs about factors that prevented them from cooperating with therapeutic procedures have been explored, the therapist can then focus the consultation on strategies for getting around the blocks with questions like these.

- *Do you think there are any ways around these obstacles?*
- *What would you need to be able to do it?*
- *What do you think Francis would have to do first before she could feel comfortable about finishing this task?*
- *Who would you need to talk to in the wider family to sort this out, so you would be free to go ahead and solve the problem?*
- *Is there any way you believe that your partner could find the courage to follow through on this, even though its a big threat to him?*
- *It sounds like the task I invited you to do was just too hard. Can you suggest an easier one that would get you to where you want to go?*

The pros and cons of any course of action that work around resistances may be explored using the following sorts of questions.

- *Who would be most put out by this new plan?*
- *Even if you could do this, there would be a price to be paid. I don't know if that's something you are ready to do?*
- *What is the cloud that goes with this silver lining? Can you put up with this cloud for a while?*

When resistance has been questioned and ways around it explored, the last step is to frame the therapeutic dilemma. This is a statement of the costs of maintaining the status quo as against the price of circumventing resistance and pursuing change. Here are some examples.

- *On the one hand you want to teach Charles to be honest so that he will not grow up and become a delinquent. On the other, you feel like you will be biasing the teacher against him if you meet with her regularly for a while to check on Charles homework. Both ways there is a price to pay.*
- *You want Tracy to stop starving herself. You know that if she continues she will become ill, and that one in five anorexics die. You know that its serious. But when you follow the programme here, she shouts at you and you feel like she may end up hating you. Its a difficult position.*
- *You both want what is best for David, but if you both do what you believe is best you end up arguing and David will suffer. Because Robert, you see the important thing is for him to develop independence so he needs to go to boarding school. May, you think the most important thing is for him to feel loved. So he needs to stay at home. Finding a way that he can be independent and loved is tricky, because you will have to negotiate about that. But in both of your families where you grew up, it was a sign of weakness for fathers to negotiate with mothers. What the men said was what happened. So, if you negotiate, both of you, but particularly you, Robert, will feel like you are being weak. This will lead you to become angry with May. A fight will occur and David will suffer. This is a difficult dilemma.*

FIVE FACTORS CONTRIBUTING TO RESISTANCE

In the previous section it was mentioned that five main types of factors underpin most resistance to co-operating with the consultation process:

1. Unpredictable events (Acts of God)
2. Lack of ability
3. Lack of commitment

4. Beliefs related to the problem
5. Emotional pain.

Preliminary ways of inquiring about these factors have been outlined already. In this section each factor will be explored in some detail.

Acts of God

Sometimes, failure to complete a task can occur because of an unforeseen change in a client's circumstances: an Act of God. This is the case in the following example.

Over a series of six sessions, two fosterparents failed to complete the tasks necessary to achieve the goal of helping a teenage fosterchild on short term placement complete an evening meal without engaging in verbally-abusive conflict. The failure was, in large part, associated with the erratic and stormy series of unscheduled and unforeseen visits that occurred between the fosterchild and his natural parents during the period in which the therapy was occurring. The relationship between poor therapeutic progress and the visits was an important therapeutic focus in the sixth session. The way in which the visits activated the teenager's sense of insecurity and his ambivalent feelings about both the fosterparents and his natural parents was explored. Management of the resistance focused on developing a strategy with the social worker and the teenager's natural parents for arranging a more predictable schedule of visits.

Lack of Ability

If failure to make progress is due to mismatch between clients' abilities or skills and the tasks they are invited to carry out, then a new goal consistent with the clients' ability levels must be set. A common error, illustrated by the next example, is to assume that clients have the micro-skills necessary to complete macro-assignments. In these cases, coaching in skill development in the session may be necessary, or more modest intersession tasks need to be set.

Members of a chaotic distressed family with a handicapped child set the goal of having a weekly family outing. They consistently failed to achieve this goal because they lacked the communication skills or conflict management skills necessary to plan the outing without serious conflict occurring. This goal was put on the backburner, and an intermediate goal introduced which was more consistent with their ability level: to complete an active listening assignment on a weekly basis for a month.

Lack of Commitment

Resistance may also be due to lack of commitment to the consultation process. This type of resistance occurs when a good contract for therapy has not been established or when an engagement mistake has been made. Methods for establishing therapy contracts are discussed in Chapter 7. Engagement mistakes are described in Chapter 2. In multiproblem cases a common therapeutic mistake is to select a goal to which the therapist is committed but to which the client is not. For example, a therapist selected improving family communication as a primary goal, whereas the parents were adamant that getting better housing was their main priority.

Exploration of resistance due to lack of commitment involves asking the customer question mentioned first in Chapter 4:

• *Who is most concerned about the problem?*

Beliefs

Specific beliefs, relevant to the presenting problem, may trap family members into a particular role in the pattern of interaction around the presenting problem. These beliefs may prevent family members from engaging in new behaviours or therapeutic tasks that may liberate them from the pattern of interaction around the presenting problem. In was noted in Chapter 3, that these beliefs (which are placed in the middle column of a three column formulation model) may have their roots in family members' life scripts, family myths or cultural norms.

In managing resistance associated specifically with clients' belief systems, Cronen and Pearce's (1985) model for analysing social behaviour is particularly useful.

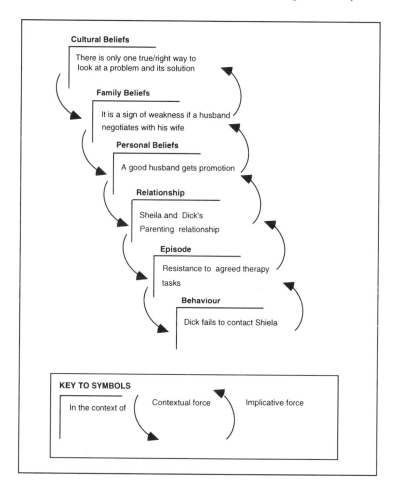

Figure 11.2.   Analysis of beliefs contributing to resistance using Cronen and Pearce's framework

This model provides a framework for planning lines of inquiry and for organizing the sets of client beliefs that emerge from such lines of questioning. You will remember that in the fourth session with the Barrows, I asked Caroline and Sheila a series of questions about beliefs underpinning Dick's difficulty in co-operating with the therapeutic task of providing Sheila with daily support in relation to her care of Caroline. The results of this line of inquiry are presented in Figure 11.2. Cronen and Pearce's model has been used to organize the material. The model views any behaviour as occurring within the context of an episode. Each episode occurs within the context of a relationship. Behaviour within a relationship occurs within the context of individual belief systems or scripts. These in turn evolve within the context of family belief systems. Family belief systems evolve within a cultural context. When Dick did not cooperate with the therapeutic task, his behaviour was determined to some degree by each of the contextual forces diagrammed in Figure 11.2 and this behaviour in turn had an implicative impact on the episode, the relationship, Dick's beliefs and so forth.

When Cronen and Pearce's model is used to plan lines of inquiry, it directs the therapist to ask questions about the impact of beliefs at each contextual level on the resistant behaviour. Here are some simple examples, each of which could be followed up with probes.

- *X agreed to do Y but something stopped this happening. What personal beliefs that X holds do you think stopped him?*
- *In X's family, what beliefs that his parents/grandparents/ siblings hold would have prevented him from doing Y?*
- *What deep belief that X holds as an English person/Irish person/Catholic/Traveller prevented him from doing Y?*

For clients to be able to cooperate with therapeutic tasks, the tasks must be consistent with beliefs at all levels of Cronen and Pearce's model. The three options for action suggested to Dick in the letter presented in Figure 11.1 were designed to be consistent with his individual life script, his family belief system and with cultural norms.

Where it is not possible to co-construct solutions consistent with clients' core beliefs, therapy must focus on helping clients to reinterpret cultural norms, family myths or personal life scripts. However, this is often emotionally painful and extremely time-consuming. In Positive Practice, which has been developed as a brief approach to therapy for child-focused problems, this line of action is only taken when other avenues are blocked. However, a proportion of parents at the end of an episode of child-focused work may recontract for individual or marital therapy to address personal, family-of-origin or cultural script issues.

Emotional Pain

The fifth factor underpinning resistance is emotional pain. Many parents resist cooperating with the therapist when they see that the resolution of the child's symptoms may entail them making difficult changes in their own lives. They begin to sense the emotional pain that goes with making these changes. Taking responsibility for making these changes often means negotiating new roles; dealing with the risk of anger, disapproval or fear that will occur in these negotiations; developing new skills and facing the risk of failure in doing so; or giving up cherished beliefs about the self and others and mourning the loss of these. All of these processes entail emotional pain: pain which the therapist cannot magically undo or soothe. Clients try to avoid this pain in a variety of ways. These include claiming to be a powerless victim and therefore unable to change; projecting responsibility for the problem and its resolution into one person or agency and blaming them for not changing; or avoiding the problem by distracting the focus of the therapeutic conversation away from the problem and its resolution. Let us examine these expressions of resistance in more detail.

HELPLESSNESS, BLAMING AND DISTRACTION AS EXPRESSIONS OF RESISTANCE

Helplessness

Clients may simply stay stuck and make no move to take on the responsibility for change which has shifted onto their shoulders. In these cases, invitations to take on therapeutic tasks are not taken up. Consultations become sterile whinging sessions where problems are endlessly described and clients berate themselves endlessly for being impotent to change their circumstances. This is usually done with good reason. Such clients' beliefs in their own powerlessness are typically based on a long history of failure in dealing with a variety of issues, including the current presenting problem. Many such clients are depressed and exhibit all the hallmarks of what Martin Seligman has termed the Learned Helplessness Syndrome (Abramson, Seligman and Teasdale, 1978). The commonest countertransference reaction to helplessness is to alternate between rescuing and persecuting. That is, therapists move from a position where they have been taking too much responsibility for the clients' problems to one where they criticise the client for not taking responsibility. Here are some questions that may be asked when faced with this resistance.

- *Let us pretend for a few minutes that you had a little power. Not a lot. Just a little. And you only had one chance to use it. Like a prisoner escaping with one bullet in her gun. How would you use this single shot of power to sort your problem out? How do you think other family members would use their single shot of power?*
- *I notice that you talk about yourself as powerless to change your situation. But I have watched you do some very powerful things like accepting a referral, agreeing to a treatment contract and dealing with the housing people. My guess is that you think that something bad will happen if you start to try to use more and more of this power. I'm wondering what that is?*
- *Powerlessness has caught you in her web. But one time you were free. Tell me about that time? What was the difference between that time and this? What would you need to do to get to a place where you were free from this web of powerlessness?*

Blaming

Another tack that clients take when they find taking on responsibility for changing their own circumstances painful is to blame other people (including the therapist) for not rescuing them. In some such cases the parents use sessions as a forum for mutual criticism. In others, one child is selected to be the scapegoat for the family difficulties, and sessions are used to criticise and blame this individual for all the family's problems. The family may alternatively choose to criticise grandparents, friends, fosterparents, the school, the social worker, the probation officer, the housing authority or any other involved agency singly or collectively for their difficulties. It is easy for the therapist to collude with this blaming for many reasons. First, there is always a grain of truth in the criticisms, and unsupported or stressed therapists may wish to indulge themselves in blaming some aspect of the system for the lack of progress, rather than accept that they have failed to help the family make therapeutic progress. Second, most therapists collude with blaming because they sense unconsciously that if they point out that blaming is being used by clients to avoid taking responsibility for problem resolution, the clients will transfer the blame to the therapist. Here are some useful questions to use when resistance takes the form of blaming. This question invites behavioural change without exploring the beliefs that underpin the blaming.

- *This is the formulation of the problem that we have all accepted. (Point to the formulation on the board.) Everyone plays a part in maintaining this problem. At the moment it seems important for you to blame your wife, the school and possibly me for not resolving the difficulties described here. Now these criticisms may all be valid. But what I am inviting you to do is this. To think about what can you do now to change your part in this formulation. Maybe this is something that you would rather do than blaming. I don't know?*

The following question aims to uncover the beliefs that underpin the blaming.

- *None of us like to be blamed, yet we all do it. We do it most when we know there is something we should do but we are frightened if we do that something bad will happen. What bad thing do you think will happen if you/your husband / your wife / your child does something to sort this problem out rather than blaming other people?*

Distracting

Sometimes, clients avoid taking responsibility for changing their situation by distracting the therapist or other members of the family from the central objective of therapy: resolving the presenting problem. Distraction can take many forms. In some cases—*the cocktail party syndrome*—one or more family members simply talk a lot about irrelevant material and no one can get a word in edgeways. For example, the father of a family with an obsessive child shared a keen interest in sailing with me. He would gladly have spent entire sessions discussing boats and sailboards rather than looking at ways to help his son resolve his obsessive-compulsive problems.

In other cases—*where intellectualizing occurs*—one or more family members talk endlessly about relevant material but in an intellectual way. A teacher with an interest in English literature and psychoanalysis, whose daughter was referred with hysterical fainting fits, talked incessantly to me about her psychoanalytic interpretations of her daughter's fits, but had great difficulty focusing on helping her daughter learn to control the fainting spells.

A third form of distraction—*the red herring*—is where some member of the family tries to lure the therapist into an irrelevant area with new symptoms. A teenager referred for solvent abuse, any time she relapsed, would begin the session by describing some vivid frightening dream and asking for an interpretation.

A fourth form of distraction—*the free for all*—is where all family members talk at once, either to each other or to the therapist. In one blended multiproblem family, with six children and four parents referred because all of the children had various conduct problems, it took two sessions to establish a contract for assessment because all family members always talked simultaneously, and wandered in and out of the session to have cigarettes, take children to the toilet or gossip in the corridor.

There are many other forms of distraction that occur where clients will talk about anything except their difficulty in taking action to resolve the presenting problem. In all of these, the overriding therapeutic task is to refocus the conversation on problem resolution and to reintroduce the rule that no one person may dominate the conversation and everybody must listen to the person who is talking.

One non-verbal technique that is particularly useful in establishing turntaking is to use the *conch*. In Golding's *Lord of the Flies,* in meetings of the council, members were only allowed to speak if they held a large sea shell which symbolised authority: the conch. This practice is also useful in family therapy. The rules of turn-taking need to be clearly spelled out. Everybody gets a turn. When it is their turn they hold the conch and speak. No one can interrupt except the therapist, if they speak for more than four minutes. When a person has finished talking they hand the conch back to the therapist who then passes it to the person whose turn it is next.

The following questions may be used to refocus the conversation away from distracting or irrelevant themes.

- *What you have said interests me. Its the sort of thing I'd love to talk about for a while, but my job is to help you find a way out of this mess. So let's move on to talking about that. Let's start by looking at how the homework went.*
- *You know I'm really interested in that stuff. So every week you come in and talk to me about it and then I notice that I've let you down. I've spent half of your time gossiping when I should have been working. So lets get down to work straightaway today?*
- *Just say we spent less time talking about the problem in an intellectual way and more time talking about what you could do to change it, what would be the most threatening thing about that?*

NEUTRALITY, CURIOSITY AND COUNTERTRANSFERENCE

The therapeutic stance from which resistance is questioned and explored must be one of neutral curiosity rather than censure or blame. Most therapists experience some disappointment, anger or frustration when clients do not follow through on tasks that they have agreed to complete, when they fail to turn up to appointments or where they insist on prolonging therapy unnecessarily.

This type of countertransference reaction is understandable. To use Karpman's framework (which is set out in Figure 10.6), inside every therapist there is a *rescuer* who derives self-esteem from saving the client/*victim* from some *persecuting* force. When the victim refuses to be rescued or insists on being endlessly rescued, the therapist may find that an emotional urge to persecute emerges. Elsewhere I termed this countertransference reaction—*persecuting the family* (Carr, 1989).

The origin of this urge to rescue is complex and unique to each of us. A consistent theme, however, among helping professionals is the need to rescue others as a symbolic way of rescuing some archaic vulnerable aspect of themselves. This aspect of the self often owes its genesis to the experience of some unmet childhood need. Indeed, the value of personal therapy as part of therapists' continuing professional development is that it allows us to gain insight into these intrapsychic dynamics and work through them so that we are freer to take a neutral and curious stance when dealing with our clients' resistances.

Countertransference reactions may be sparked off, not only by clients' difficulties in following through on therapeutic tasks, therapy attendance and termination but by personal characteristics or the types of problems with which they present. Some therapists may find that they are particularly attracted to rescuing the women and children in families and to persecuting the males. Others may find that this pattern of countertransference only occurs in families where a bereavement has occurred, or where delinquency is the presenting problem. Families where child abuse has occurred elicit strong countertransference reactions in all of us (Carr, 1989). Four of these deserve particular mention.

In cases of physical child abuse the two commonest countertransference reactions are *rescuing the child* and *rescuing the parents*. In the former reaction, the urge is to protect the child at all costs and to deny any loyalty that the child may have to the parents, or any competence or potential for therapeutic change on the part of the parents. In the latter reaction the urge is to protect the parents from criticism raised by other professionals, and to deny any parental shortcomings. Professionals within the same system adopting these two countertransference reactions tend to polarise and have difficulty cooperating with each other and the family with whom they are working. We will return to a discussion of the impact of countertransference reactions on the cooperation of professionals within a network in Chapter 15.

In cases of intrafamilial child sexual abuse *rescuing the father* is one common countertransference reaction. The other is *rescuing the mother and child while persecuting the father*. The first reaction leads therapists to deny evidence pointing to the father's culpability and to highlight the father's strengths as a parent. The second reaction is associated with an urge to split the father off from the rest of the family and to deny any loyalties that other members may have to him. These two countertransference reactions are complimentary, and professionals experiencing them may tend to polarise each other, thus compromising their ability to work cooperatively in the service of the clients.

If therapists act out their countertransference reactions they become part of the cycle of interaction surrounding the presenting problem. That is, they become part of a behaviour pattern that maintains rather than resolves the presenting difficulties. The therapist's emotionally driven aggressive or protective behaviour fails to help family members evolve new belief systems and new ways of behaving in relation to the presenting problem. This is illustrated in Figure 11.3. In this figure a hypothesis about the impact of acting out aggressive countertransference reactions to the Barrow family is outlined. Where therapists retain a neutral and therapeutically curious position, they offer opportunities for clients to evolve new belief systems and to develop alternatives to becoming stuck in the pattern of interaction around the presenting problem.

SUMMARY

Clients show resistance in a wide variety of ways. In family consultations resistance may take the form of not completing tasks between sessions, not attending sessions, or refusing to terminate the therapy process. It may also involve not co-operating during therapy sessions. For clients to make progress with the resolution of their difficulties the therapist must have some systematic way of dealing with resistance.

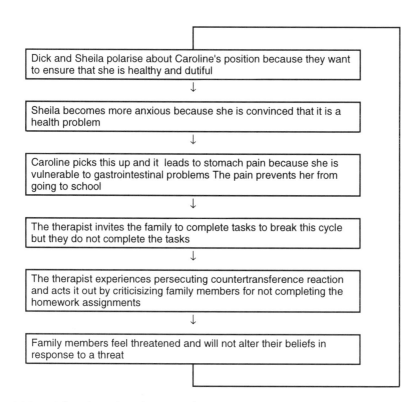

Figure 11.3. A hypothesis about the impact of acting out a persecuting countertransference reaction in the Barrow case

In Positive Practice the following step-by-step process is used. First describe the discrepancy between what clients agreed to do and what they actually did. Second, ask about the difference between situations where they managed to follow through on an agreed course of action and those where they did not. Third, ask what they believed blocked them from making progress. Fourth, ask if these blocks can be overcome. Fifth, ask about strategies for getting around the blocks. Sixth, ask about the pros and cons of these courses of action. Seventh, frame a therapeutic dilemma which outlines the costs of maintaining the status quo and the costs of circumventing the blocks.

When resistance is questioned, factors that underpin are uncovered. In some instances unforeseen events -Acts of God- hinder progress. In others the problem is that the clients lack the skills and abilities that underpin resistance. Where a poor therapy contract has been formed or an engagement mistake has been made, resistance is usually due to a lack of commitment to the therapeutic process. Specific convictions which form part of clients' individual, family or culturally based belief systems may also contribute to resistance. The wish to avoid emotional pain is a further factor that commonly underpins resistance.

Questioning resistance is only helpful if the therapist adopts a position characterised by neutrality and curiosity. If clients feel that they are being blamed for not making progress, then they will usually respond by pleading helplessness, blaming the therapist or someone else for the resistance, or distracting the focus of therapy away from the problem of resistance into less painful areas. Distraction may take a number of forms including the cocktail party syndrome, intellectualising, mentioning red herrings or treating the session as a free for all.

Blaming, distraction or pleading helplessness often elicit countertransference reactions on the therapist's part which compound rather than resolve the therapeutic impasse. The commonest of these is persecuting the family. In cases of physical child abuse therapists often adopt one of two countertransference reactions: rescuing the child or rescuing the parents. In cases of intrafamilial sexual abuse rescuing the father is a common countertransference reaction as is its counterpart: rescuing the mother and child and persecuting the father. These two pairs of countertransference reactions, common in cases of physical and sexual child abuse, lead to polarization among professionals and compromise the process of problem resolution and the quest for viable solutions. They are discussed in more detail in Chapter 15.

Exercise 11.1.

Work in pairs taking therapist and client roles.

The client must select a decision that he or she will have to make in the next 12 months.

The therapist must help the client list the pros and cons of making a decision that leads to noticeable life changes and the pros and cons of maintaining the status quo.

Swap roles and repeat the exercise.

1. Write down the three main things that you noticed about the situation when you were taking the client role.

2. Identify those two aspects of interviewing that you found relatively easy and those which you found challenging.

Exercise 11. 2.

The following four exercises are based on the Stuart case, which we first came across in Chapter 4 and around which the exercises in Chapters 8, 9 and 10 were based. You will remember that Paul Stuart is aged 9 and was referred by the GP who identified encopresis, attainment problems and disobedience at home as the main problems. A three column formulation of the case is given at the end of Chapter 8.

Work in groups of at least 6 members. Five people take the roles of members of the Stuart family. The remaining person or people take the roles of the therapist and team. You must plan and conduct an interview in which you explore resistance. The family have not completed a task you invited them to carry out in a previous session. You must agree what this task was before the exercise begins. You may base the task on ideas you generated in Exercise 9.1.

The family members must take ten minutes to get into role, and work out an agreed chain of events that and circumstances associated with the resistance. Then, participate in the interview for 10 minutes.

Derole after the interview.

Take 20 minutes to discuss

1.   What the experience was like for family members and
2.   Which aspects of the interviewing process were within the therapist's competence and
        which offered the greatest challenge.

12

Written Communication

Written communication has an important role in Positive Practice. Letters may be used to help clients remember what was said during consultation, and to highlight key aspects of the sessions. Letters also provide a medium for involving other members of the system in the therapeutic process, including absent family members, the referring agent and involved professionals. Letters may be used creatively as a medium for reframing problems. Correspondence between family members may be encouraged to help family members change roles. Children may be invited to engage in correspondence with imaginary characters as a way of receiving new ideas about how to change their situation. Finally, letters may be used to tell youngsters parables which may offer them a different perspective on how to cope with difficulties. Let us look at each of these ways of using letters in Positive Practice in more detail.

LETTERS AS AIDS TO MEMORY

Any aspect of the consultation process may be recapped in a letter. Here, the function of the letter is to help family members remember what has happened in the session. Thus letters can be used to give family members a written account of the formulation, a summary of what has taken place in a session, details of the contract for therapy, a reframing of some aspect of their problem, a summary of tasks they have been invited to complete or administrative information about appointments, other relevant services, and so forth. One aspect of this use of letters has already been mentioned in Chapter 9, where it was noted that families are more likely to complete tasks if the tasks are written down.

The Clanwilliam Institute
Clanwilliam Terrace
Dublin

Dr Brannigan
The Surgery
Main Street
Greystones

9.2.93

Re: Kim O'Byrne (DOB 7.8.79) The Cottage, Greystones

Dear Dr Brannigan

We spoke about Kim on the phone last week and I met with Kim and her parents today for the first time. I have nothing to add to the extensive history that you gave me on the phone. The O'Byrnes have a track record of being a well functioning family. The main noteworthy feature concerns Mrs Mary O'Byrne. She had panic attacks with agoraphobia for about five years, but she overcame her problems through psychotherapy and behaviour modification about ten years ago.

Kim's development and adjustment were all well within normal limits up until she found the ritualistically murdered donkey last August. From her current presentation and the way she describes the past four months, she qualifies for a diagnosis of Post-Traumatic Stress Disorder (what used to be called War Neurosis). For Kim, finding the dead animal was a major stress. First, because the animal was her special pet, and second, because caring for animals generally is a major part of her value system. Since August she has continually reexperienced the horror of the event. She finds that intrusive thoughts, vivid images and intense feelings related to the event occur when she is awake and her sleep is broken by nightmares.

The problem is compounded by confusion within the family about how to cope with it. Kim believes that she has caused her parents enough trouble and so tries not to talk about the intrusive thoughts, images and feelings of anxiety or nightmares. Her mother encourages her to talk about it, because she knows from her own experience of counselling that a problem shared is a problem halved. When Kim refuses to talk, Pat, the father, encourages Kim to distract herself or suppress the feelings, a coping strategy that worked for him when he was in the army. Of course, this only works in the short term and as bedtime approaches each day the feelings intensify and anxiety about the nightmares recur. Kim takes a long time to go to sleep and then the cycle starts again when she wakes in the small hours of the morning following a nightmare.

I have enclosed a diagram of this formulation of the problem with this note.

In my opinion the key to the problem is first to help the O'Byrnes understand this formulation. Then, in the light of this, to decide upon a more effective coping strategy that all three of them can buy into. I will discourage distraction and suppression. This clearly makes things worse. I will encourage Kim to seek regular daily opportunities to ventilate her feelings with her mother. In addition, to give Kim a sense of control over the nightmares, I will train her to use self-hypnosis to revisualize her dreams and change the endings so that they become humorous or absurd rather than frightening. This is a strategy that has worked successfully for other youngsters with PTSD.

Once again, many thanks for the referral.

Dr Alan Carr

Figure 12.1.   Letter to Dr Brannigan about the O'Byrnes

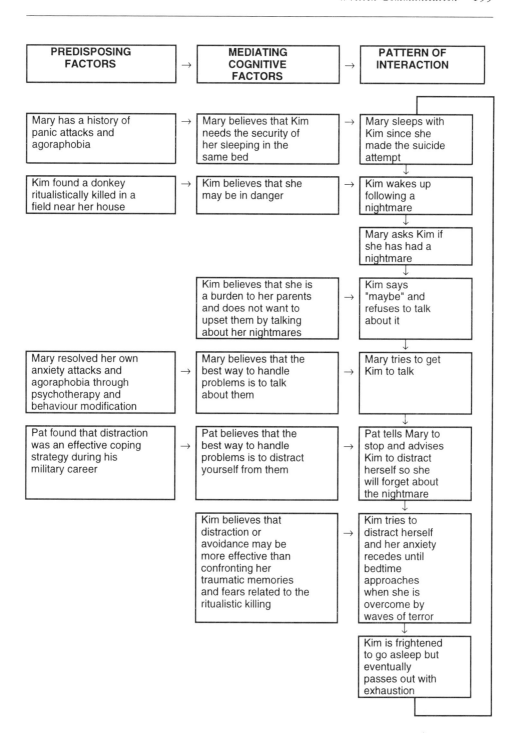

Figure 12.2.   Formulation for the O'Byrnes

LETTERS AS A WAY OF INCLUDING THE REFERRER IN THE CONSULTATION PROCESS

In Positive Practice therapists' letters are usually written to the referring agent to explain both the formulation and the direction the consultation process will take. Sufficient detail must be given so that the referring agent's interaction with the clients will facilitate rather than hinder problem resolution. In Figure 12.1 my letter to the GP who referred Kim O'Byrne explains how her post-traumatic stress disorder evolved and how it was being maintained by the family's attempts to cope with Kim's nightmares and intrusive thoughts and feelings. The therapy plan is also outlined which involves all members of the problem-system accepting ventilation of feelings rather than suppression of them as the best strategy for helping Kim recover from the trauma. The letter implicitly provides guidelines for the GP's interaction with family members should they visit him for other reasons and bring up this problem in conversation. The formulation for the case is also appended to the letter in diagrammatic form. This is presented in Figure 12.2.

LETTERS AS A METHOD FOR INCLUDING ABSENT MEMBERS IN THE SESSION

Sometimes, important family members cannot attend a consultation. For example, following the third session with the Barrow family, which Dick could not attend, you will recall that I wrote to him as a way of including him in the session and eliciting his views on how to manage the problem of offering Sheila support. This letter is contained in Figure 11.1.

On another occasion, I wrote to the father of a child whose parents were separated, asking for his views on how the next access visit should be arranged. The mother had custody of the boy and lived in Norfolk. The father lived a few hundred miles north in Scotland. The boy's loyalty was divided between his mother and father and he was unable to commit himself to spending the Easter break with his father. My letter to the father, Mr Frank Levine, is contained in Figure 12.3 and Frank's reply which was used in a later therapy session is presented in Figure 12.4. The letter from Frank freed Harry to make a decision to visit him with the proviso that he could come home a few days early if he felt disloyal to his mother. This example illustrates how letters may be used as a way of including distant family members in the consultation process.

REFRAMING LETTERS

All letters affect the way in which clients construe the presenting problem. But in Positive Practice some letters are designed with the expressed intention of co-constructing with the client a new way of looking at the problem situation. The letter in Figure 12.5 was sent to the parents of an encopretic boy who were seen briefly at the request of a paediatrician for a consultation which was interrupted before a formulation or reframing could be given. The eleven year old was referred with a five month history of soiling. His parents were interpreting the soiling as veiled aggression. This way of making sense of the encopresis was informed by a television documentary which they

```
                                    Child and Family Clinic
                                    Market Town
                                    Norfolk
Mr Frank Levine
15 Charlestown Road
Portlethen
Scotland
                                    20.3.90

Dear Frank

Harry was referred to me recently by Dr Connors, the GP. He has been having nightmares and
some problems with bullying at school. The bullying has been taken care of, but the nightmares
continue. They seem to be related to a dilemma he faces this Easter.

Recently, he has said that he is in two minds about spending all of his Easter holidays in Scotland.
On the one hand, he really wants to see you and spend as much time with you as possible because
he misses you a lot. On the other, he does not want to make his mother feel lonely by staying
away too long. Marion, as you know, is happy for him to spend the full two weeks with you.
However, Harry fears that you will be angry if he needs to come home a few days early. This is
worrying him so much, that sometimes he doubts if he should go at all and gets these bad dreams.

I cannot make a judgement about whether it would be in his best interests to go without your views.
It would help me to help your son manage his nightmares if you would write an open letter that we
can read in the next consultation giving your view on these matters.

I look forward to hearing from you.

Yours sincerely

Dr Alan Carr
```

Figure 12.3.   A letter to Frank Levine about his son's nightmares

```
                                    15 Charlestown Road
                                    Portlethen
                                    Scotland
Dr Carr
Child and Family Clinic
Market Town
Norfolk
                                    28.3.90

Dear Dr Carr

Harry should not be afraid to visit me. I want him to stay two weeks here. I have a new fishing rod
for him and I hope that we can do that big trip we always planned. But if he has to go home to see
his mother, I will not argue. I have told Marion this before but she doesn't believe me. I will not
argue and Harry must understand that.

Our visits have always been good. The last time he was here we went to the lake nearly every day.

I am sorry that he was bullied in school. He needs a man to show him how to defend himself. I will
show him some judo when he comes up to visit.

Tell Harry, that I will phone him soon.

Yours Sincerely

Frank Levine
```

Figure 12.4.   Frank Levine's reply to the letter about nightmares

had seen. The letter offers a plausible reframing of the soiling as a conditioned response to an anal fissure compounded by the later use of laxatives. Responsibility for the symptom is taken away from the boy and the parents, through this essentially mechanical reframing of the problem. This letter was pivotal in changing the way in which the parents, Barry and Sally, viewed their son, Bernard. In the second session which followed the receipt of the letter, the quality of the parent-child relationships had changed radically. Discussion focused on the implications of the reframing of the problem presented in the letter. The aggression, hostility and resentment which precluded negotiation and problem-solving in the first session dissipated. With much humour and good will the family responded to my suggestion that an enema be arranged, in conjunction with the referring paediatrician, to remove the faecal mass, and that this be followed up with a simple star chart programme.

LETTERS TO FACILITATE ROLE CHANGE

Letters can be used explicitly to facilitate changes in family members' roles. Brian, a seventeen year old, was referred with headaches which were interfering with his study

---

                                                    Child and Family Clinic
                                                    Market Town
                                                    Norfolk

Mr Tom and Sally Redwick
Little Snoring
Norfolk

Dear Barry and Sally

You asked today if Bernard was soiling because he didn't want to grow up. You speculated that he wanted to remain a baby like Caris. You guessed that the soiling was his way of being angry at your attempts to encourage him to grow up. That is one viewpoint. There is no denying that. There is another possibility. It is complicated but it seems to fit with the information I got from the GP this afternoon.

(1) Bernard unfortunately developed an anal fissure a year ago. A sore bottom. Anytime he tried to go to the toilet it was very painful. So, his unconscious told him not to. It said "Don't go to the toilet. Its too painful".
(2) When he didn't go for a while he got all blocked up. He developed a big faecal mass in his lower intestines and colon.
(3) Then you gave him a laxative. This melted the edge of the mass and it dribbled out.
(4) There was a fight about this and Bernard got anxious and his unconscious said to him "Don't go to the toilet. it only leads to trouble".
The faecal mass grew even bigger
(5) The process repeated again and again.

This process is nobody's fault. Just an unfortunate situation. I've spoken to the Paediatrician, Dr Connors, who will be happy to check the state of Bernard's faecal mass and advise on how best to get rid of it. After that we can develop a plan to prevent this happening again. You will hear from the Paediatrics Department shortly.

Yours sincerely

Dr Alan Carr

Figure 12.5.   A letter used to reframe Bernard's encopresis

and with his sports. The headaches occurred when he overheard his parents arguing. His parents, both articulate and fiery characters, resolved their differences through loud and dramatic arguments in which crockery was occasionally broken. As part of therapy I helped the parents, Sharon and Trevor, compose the letter in Figure 12.6. They read it out to Brian after supper, at my suggestion, and asked him to keep it on the notice board in his room as a reminder that the arguments were a sign of commitment rather than impending divorce.

Brian

We know that you have been worrying about us arguing.
We are sorry that the worry causes you to have headaches.
We want you to stop worrying so your headaches will go away.

We want you to know that when we argue, this does not mean that we are going to separate. It means that we have different opinions and we need to talk about that. Arguing is a sign that we care about each other. We need to argue with each other from time to time.

If you don't like the sound of us arguing we will not be offended if you listen to your walkman or go out for a walk.

Thank you for worrying about us but now you deserve a break from it.

Mum and Dad

Figure 12.6.   A letter from Sharon and Trevor to their teenager Brian

LETTERS FROM IMAGINARY AUTHORS

Occasionally, I have enlisted the aid of imaginary authors in the treatment of children. Bozz is one of my favourite. He is an expert at helping youngsters *Boss their Hammermen about*. When children have temper control difficulties and routine behavioural control programmes have not worked or the parents oppose such approaches, the aggressive impulses are personified as the *Hammerman* or some other character. The child is then given advice on how to control the hammerman from Bozz, a fictitious character with whom they find it easy to identify. They are encouraged to develop a correspondence with him. A letter from Bozz to Tom Holden, an eight year old boy referred with temper control problems, is contained in Figure 12.7. This is just one part of an ongoing correspondence which lasted six weeks. The use of imaginary authors like Bozz allows the therapist to adopt a position where he or she can comment to the youngster and the parents about the correspondence their child is having with Bozz.

PARABLES

The use of parables, myths and fairy tales to help people find solutions to problems of living is a custom that has its roots in the oral storytelling tradition. Within the family therapy field, Milton Erickson has played a major part in the integration of this ancient

```
┌────────────────────────────────────────────────────────────────────────┐
│                                                        Bozz's Place       │
│ Tom Holden                                                                │
│ Hunstanton                                                                │
│ Norfolk                                                                   │
│                                                                           │
│ Dear Tom                                                                  │
│                                                                           │
│ I know that you want to keep the hammerman from getting you into trouble. So here is what you │
│ can do. You can take him down to the end of the garden every morning at 8.15 before school and │
│ every evening at 4.00 and get him to whack the tennis ball against the wall until he's too tired to do │
│ any more. If he tries to get you into trouble with your sister say to him │
│ **Hammerman hold it!**                                                     │
│ If you can't control him, ask your mum if you can go down to the end of the garden and let │
│ hammerman whack the ball up against the wall.                              │
│                                                                           │
│ Write and tell me how you got on.                                         │
│                                                                           │
│ Bozz                                                                      │
└────────────────────────────────────────────────────────────────────────┘
```

Figure 12.7.   A letter from Bozz to Tom about Hammerman

tradition into modern clinical practice (Haley, 1973). The key to using parables in a clinical situation is to take the salient elements of the client's situation and build them into a story which arrives at a conclusion that offers the client an avenue for productive change rather than a painful cul-de-sac. The story is a metaphor for the client's dilemma, a metaphor that offers a solution. Such stories may be sent to clients as letters. The story contained in Figure 12.9 was sent to, Sabina, a seven year old girl who was referred because of recurrent nightmares in which she dreamt that her house was being burgled and her parents assaulted. The nightmares followed an actual burglary of the family's shop, over which they lived. The girl dealt with the nightmares by climbing onto the end of her parents bed when she awoke at night. She tried not to wake them and distracted herself by thinking of something other than the nightmares. During the day she refused to talk about the nightmares or the burglary. To some degree, her parents encouraged this process of denial. Sabina was in the brownies and was learning about first aid when she was referred. Towards the end of the first session I offered the story set out in Figure 12.8 and subsequently sent it to Sabina with the letter contained in Figure 12.9.

This story took account of Sabina's interest in first aid and racing. A physical trauma (cutting her knee) was used as a metaphor for the psychological trauma she had suffered (being burgled). The story included one course of action taken by the dark haired girl which resembled the pattern of coping she had adopted. It also contained an alternative. This other more adaptive route was taken by the blond girl; the girl whose hair was the same colour as Sabina's. This detail was included to make it easy for Sabina to identify with her. The story reframed Sabina's dilemma from "How can I distract myself from memories of the robbery and get rid of these nightmares so I can feel good?" to "How can I squeeze all of this psychological pus out of my mind so the wound will heal?" This reframing offered a new avenue for coping.

The Two Brownies

Two brownies were on an adventure in the woods. They decided to have a race. They were both the same height and looked alike except that one had blond hair like yours and one had dark hair. While they were racing they both tripped over the same branch at the same time and each of them cut their knee. The cuts hurt a lot and both girls felt like crying. The dark haired girl tried to stop herself from crying and her leg hurt more. The blond girl allowed herself to cry and felt relieved. The crying made her knee hurt less. Both girls went to the stream and bathed their cuts. Both girls had small first aid kits in their pockets. The dark haired girl put a bandage from her kit on her cut straightaway. The blond girl could have done this also but she did not. She let the air get at her cut. Both girls went home for tea. After tea they went to bed. The dark haired girl couldn't sleep because the cut hurt so much. She turned on the light. She took off the bandage and noticed that the cut had become infected. It was all yellow with pus. The dark haired girl washed the cut quickly and put on another bandage over the pus. The blond girl woke in the middle of the night because her knee was hurting her. She woke her mum and her mum helped her bathe the cut in hot water to draw the pus out. This was painful, but she knew it would make her better. Three days later her cut was healed. But her friend was still wearing a bandage. Her knee still had pus in it. She still woke up in the middle of the night with the pain.

THE END

Figure 12.8.   The story of the Two Brownies

Child and Family Clinic
Market Town
Norfolk

Sabina Grey
Pott Row
Norfolk

Dear Sabina

I really liked the pictures you did today. They gave me a clear idea of the sort of stuff you have been seeing in your dreams. I like the way you draw. Just to say thank you, here is the story I told you today. If some of the words are too hard just ask your mum or dad and they will let you know what they mean. See you in two weeks.

Bye now.

Dr Alan Carr

Figure 12.9.   Letter to Sabina about her dreams

SUMMARY

In Positive Practice letters may be used to help clients remember aspects of the consultation process and as a medium for involving other members of the system in the therapeutic process including absent family members, the referring agent and involved professionals. Letters may also be used as a medium for reframing problems and for telling parables. Ritualistic correspondence between family members may be encouraged to help family members change roles. Children may be invited to engage in correspondence with imaginary characters as a way of receiving advice about how to change their situation. White and Epston's (1990) *Narrative Means to Therapeutic Ends* provides a thorough discussion of the use of written communication in brief family therapy. Weeks and L'Abate's work (1982) also contains many creative examples of how letters may be used to facilitate the therapeutic process.

Exercise 12.1.

Think of a case where recently an important family member did not attend the consultation. Write them a letter inviting them to the next session. Explain why, specifically, it is important for them to attend.

Exercise 12.2.

Write a parable for Harry Levine (referred to in Figure 12.3). The parable must offer Harry a new way of coping with his experience of divided loyalties.

13

Therapeutic Dilemmas and Crisis Phonecalls

In Chapter 11 we saw that resistance occurs when the therapist invites the family to change but the family respond by appearing to reject this invitation. Instead they plead helplessness, they blame someone else for not solving the problem, or they try to distract the therapist away from the focus of therapy. If the therapist responds by co-constructing with the family their therapeutic dilemma which states the disadvantages of the problem and the disadvantages of taking responsibility to resolve the problem, then a therapeutic crisis will often occur.

Let us recap the therapeutic dilemma which the Barrows faced. Maintaining the status quo would lead to the following disadvantages:

1. Caroline continuing to experience pain and school absence
2. Continued anxiety for Sheila about having a child with an unknown illness
3. Continued worry for Dick about having a naughty malingering child
4. A continuous low level conflict between Dick and Sheila about the nature of the problem and how to deal with it.

Seeking a solution to the problem, on the other hand, also entailed disadvantages.

1. Dick would have to put more time and effort into his relationships with Sheila and Caroline and this might compromise his promotion prospects, which would in the long term lead to him spending more time away from the family
2. If Dick and Sheila began to negotiate about how best to solve the problem their disagreement about its nature might lead to an extremely angry argument
3. If Sheila insisted on Caroline visiting the GP when she had stomach pains, an extremely angry argument between Sheila and Caroline or between Caroline and the GP might occur because Caroline thought the GP believed she was malingering
4. The GP might mistakenly give Caroline a clean bill of health and Caroline might

develop a serious medical condition for which Sheila would feel responsible (thereby replicating the difficulty that occurred with the misdiagnosis of Sheila's mother's cancer).

Between the fourth and fifth sessions the Barrows were invited to put aside two thirty minute periods to discuss this dilemma.

CRISIS PHONECALL

Ten days after the fourth consultation and five days before the next scheduled appointment there was a crisis phonecall to the clinic from Dick at 10am. He said that Caroline refused point blank to got to school. He described her as screaming her head off like a lunatic. She had bitten him on the hand. He wanted her admitted to a psychiatric unit for sedation and inpatient evaluation.

Before asking for a fuller account of the events surrounding this crisis I checked to see if Caroline or her parents were in any danger. Caroline was in her bedroom being comforted by Sheila and there appeared to be no immediate danger to any family member. With this first step completed, I encouraged Dick to give me a blow-by-blow account of the episode. Dick explained that it all started when he became angry after receiving my letter. He felt as if he was being accused of being a failure as a parent and that this was wholly untrue. He then decided to take a very active role in helping to resolve the problem. He told Sheila that he would stay home from work and insist that Caroline attend school. On the Monday morning when the phonecall occurred, he had driven Caroline to school. She refused to leave the car because she said she had a stomachache. He offered her the choice of either visiting the GP or going to school. She refused both options and told him not to be a bully. Dick said that he knew then she was either faking the stomachaches or was seriously mentally disturbed. Her behaviour was totally out of character. He tried physically to man-handle her out of the car. She went wild, screaming, punching, kicking, and finally biting him on the hand. Her face was bright red and she was crying uncontrollably. When he let her go, she dived onto the floor in the back of the car, which was a hatchback, curled up into a ball and began rocking and crooning. Dick said that the fact that she bit him and then began to croon and rock herself, confirmed for him that she was mentally ill and required hospitalization. I encouraged Dick to talk to me about the episode at some length, to express his beliefs about the causes of Caroline's behaviour and to ventilate his mixed feelings about this painful episode. However, I took care, despite his insistence, not to agree with his interpretation of the situation as evidence that his daughter was mad, and also not to agree that the solution was hospitalization and sedation.

Dick's attempt to reframe a systemic problem in individualistic terms so that he could protect himself and the other members of the system from the practical difficulties and emotional tension entailed by negotiating a workable solution with the other members of the system, is one of the hallmarks of a therapeutic crisis in systemic consultation. I told him that if Caroline was a danger to herself or other people, I would help the family make arrangements for hospitalization, but otherwise the need was for an immediate meeting of the family with other people involved in the problem, including Caroline's teacher, the GP and the school nurse.

Dick agreed to this, as did Sheila and Caroline. Caroline took the call in her room on a portable house phone. She spoke little, but agreed to attend. She said that if she were left to herself in her own room, while arrangements for the meeting were being made, she would not hurt herself or anyone else. In the light of this, Dick backed down on his demand for Caroline's hospitalization. A meeting was scheduled for Wednesday (two days later) at 4.00pm. The Barrow family and a number of involved professionals were invited. I contacted the GP, Dr Wilson, Caroline's year-head, Ms Hackett, the Education and Welfare Officer, Phil Hutchinson and the school nurse, Nurse Boyd; filled them in on the recent crisis and invited them to the meeting. I said that the goal of the meeting was to develop a plan that would allow the Barrows to feel comfortable about the management of Caroline's pain and about her return to full time school attendance.

DILEMMAS AND CRISES

A therapeutic dilemma is a concise statement of the disadvantages and difficulties associated with leaving the presenting problem unresolved and the disadvantages and risks entailed by solving the problem. It is rarely enough to say that the symptoms are bad but the prospect of change is worse. Rather, when articulating the therapeutic dilemma it is important to relate the way in which family members are trapped in the cycle of interaction around the presenting problem to their belief systems that underpin their roles in this cycle and also to note that these belief systems have roots in their personal histories, their families of origin or their membership of other systems such as work or school. It is also important to specify or give examples of the types of action that might lead to resolving the presenting problem in the future and the emotional costs of these.

Stating the therapeutic dilemma may precipitate a therapeutic crisis. If clients see that both the problem and its resolution entail emotional pain and that the responsibility for resolving the problem is largely theirs, they will experience a crisis if they believe that they have not got the personal resources to cope with the demands of this responsibility.

A therapeutic crisis does not have to occur in every case. If the responsibilities that the therapist invites clients to take on are well within their capacity to cope, then no crisis will occur. Certain types of client are less likely to experience a therapeutic crisis. Where clients have single rather than multiple problems and mild rather than severe difficulties then they are less likely to experience a therapeutic crisis. A crisis is also less likely where clients have good coping skills and where their social support network is well established.

Therapeutic crises only become a possibility when the therapeutic system becomes well and truly stuck, as in Figure 13.1. There are certain things that a therapist can do to minimize the chance of a therapeutic crisis occurring. Therapists can help clients co-construct a formulation that entails solutions which can be broken down into a number of manageable tasks. Systematic desensitization, the behavioural method for learning to cope with phobias, is a good example of this type of strategy. Here, clients are never asked to face an extremely frightening situation which would be unmanageable. Rather, they are asked to face situations of gradually increasing fearfulness and are helped to

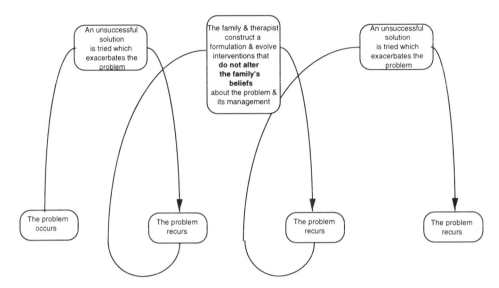

Figure 13.1.   Map of a stuck therapeutic system

cope with one before moving on to the next. The same is true of behavioural training in problem solving skills. Clients begin by being trained in how to solve emotionally neutral problems and only when they have mastered these skills are they invited to move on to tackle emotionally loaded issues relevant to the presenting problem (Falloon et al, 1993). A map of a stuck therapeutic system responding to therapy without a crisis occurring is presented in Figure 13.2.

However, in many forms of family therapy, clinicians work actively to precipitate a crisis. Salvador Minuchin, founder of Structural Family Therapy, invited families to enact their routine solutions to presenting problems in the consulting room, but encouraged family members to progress further with these solutions than they would typically go. For example, in families with anorexic teenagers, he invited the parent who saw the child as bad or disobedient and who favoured force feeding, to show him how this solution worked in practice by making the anorexic girl eat food during the consultation. When this enacted solution ended in a crisis of failure, he would invite

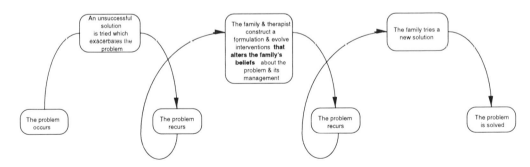

Figure 13.2.   Map of a therapeutic system responding to an intervention without a crisis

family members to consider other ways of reframing the problem and other solutions (Minuchin, Rosman and Baker, 1978). The original Milan associates precipitated family crises by articulating the necessity of the family members' roles in maintaining the presenting problem and pointing out the costs of changing the family game (Selvini Palazzoli et al, 1980). Therapeutic approaches which aim to precipitate a crisis, challenge clients to act-out or think-through their current framing of the problem and its solution. When the limitations of this are seen and the intense sadness, fear or anger associated with this realization are foreseen or experienced, clients begin to doubt their original framing of the problem (Jenkins, 1989).

In Positive Practice, where possible, therapeutic crises are avoided. However, where clients attempt new and painful solutions to difficult life problems, therapeutic crises may occur. The presentation of the therapeutic dilemma is often a catalyst which activates a family or one of its members to explore a solution entailed by the formulation or indeed, a solution entailed by their own private construction of the problem.

For example, in the Barrow case, Dick chose to disregard the three column formulation, construe Caroline as a *bad* girl who needed firm handling, and forcibly return her to school. When Caroline bit Dick and crooned in response to his treatment of her as a disobedient child, he was extremely distressed and began to doubt his framing of her as *bad* and the wisdom of the firm and ineffective approach he took in returning her to school.

In response to the doubt, he chose another simplistic individualistic framing of Caroline's behaviour. He chose to see his daughter not as *bad* but as *mad*. This is not surprising. Under stress all of us choose cognitively simple rather than complex framings of challenging or threatening situations. Also, we all choose to avoid emotionally distressing situations. When Dick reframed Caroline's difficulties as *madness* and the solution as *hospitalization and sedation* he selected a framing that would help him to avoid considerable emotional distress. By selecting an individualistic framing rather than the interactional formulation, he chose a way of conceptualizing the problem that would allow him to continue to avoid the painful process of negotiating a shared understanding of the problem with Sheila. If Caroline were *mad* then she needed expert help, *hospitalization, and sedation*. His role in the management of the problem would be peripheral. He could therefore avoid emotional pain and possibly protect Sheila from emotional pain also. He could also preserve a view of himself as a good father who was doing the best he could for his *mad* daughter.

Invariably, therapeutic crises involve some family members doubting the interactional three column formulation of the problem and redefining the problem as an individual difficulty rather than as an interactional phenomenon. That is, someone in the family becomes defined as *bad, sad, sick* or *mad* (these labels were previously noted in Chapter 10 in the discussion on individualistic belief systems and Karpman's triangle). There is usually some attempt by a member of the problem-system to convince the therapist that an individual definition of the problem is true and an interactional definition of the problem is false. Often, another professional is coopted into the system to help the family convince the therapist of the truth of the individual formulation, or to disqualify the therapists interactional formulation. This pressure to collude with the family and other network members in abandoning an interactional construction of the problem and in accepting an individual description is usually very intense. Without a framework for understanding these crises and guidelines for managing them, therapists are easily *sucked into* colluding with those members of the problem-system who wish to label one person as the problem (Selvini-Palazzoli and Prata, 1982). A map of such a stuck system is contained in Figure 13.3.

From a therapeutic point of view, the importance of a crisis is that it is a critical opportunity for change and problem resolution. Family members are faced with major difficulties about which they are extremely unclear. In Positive Practice, the therapist responds to the family's need for certainty by offering them a three column formulation as a map to guide them out of their difficulties. Fortunately, the more severe a problem is, the greater the motivation of the clients to co-operate with a therapist, provided they view the therapist as competent to help them. A map of a stuck therapeutic system responding to a therapeutic dilemma with a crisis, and the resolution of this, is presented in Figure 13.4.

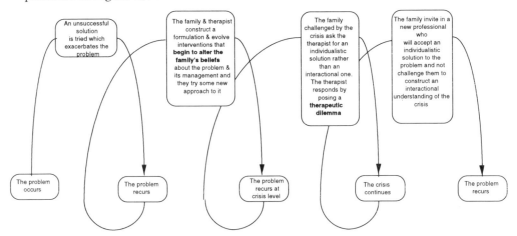

Figure 13.3.   Map of a therapeutic system responding to a therapeutic dilemma with a crisis and drawing in other professionals in a way that maintains the problem

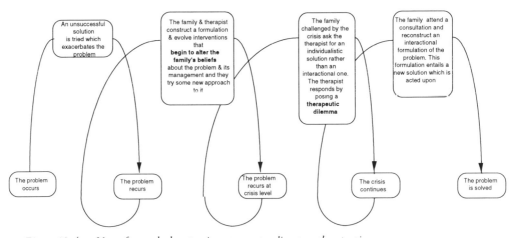

Figure 13.4.   Map of a stuck therapeutic system responding to a therapeutic dilemma with a crisis and crisis resolution

GUIDELINES FOR MANAGING THERAPEUTIC CRISES

The overriding goal in managing a therapeutic crisis is to help clients retain an interactional construction of the problem which opens up possibilities for achieving their long term therapeutic goals. By implication this involves avoiding collusion with an individualistic construction of the problem which would lead to short term relief but hinder long term goal attainment. What follows are guidelines for dealing with crises. They are framed *as if* the crisis takes the form of a phonecall from a parent. Of course this is not always the case. Some crises occur during a consultation. Others are mentioned through letters from involved professionals. However, the majority of crises in my practice have taken the form of phonecalls from parents, and so it is in this context that the guidelines are framed.

1. Assess and manage danger

Family violence, abuse, self-injurious gestures, running away, staying out late, theft, and the discovery of substance abuse are some of the incidents that occur when a therapeutic crisis is reached. In Positive Practice the clinician's first duty is to establish if anyone in the family is a danger to themselves or to other people. If there is a high risk of danger, an immediate family consultation should be scheduled. The goal of this is to help the family manage the immediate danger.

2. Empathize with the caller's emotional pain without colluding with their simplistic solutions

Parents only make crisis calls if they perceive the demands of the situation to outweigh their capacity to cope. If their child has run away or slashed their wrists, or if their spouse has screamed at them and hit a child, they may believe that these are situations with which they cannot deal. Often, in such circumstances, patents are overwhelmed by fear, sadness or anger, and these intense emotions have compromised their capacity for clear thinking and systematic problem solving. They find themselves locked into black and white thinking, unable to tolerate the complexities or ambiguities of their problem situation. So, for example, with the Barrows, Dick saw Caroline as mentally ill and was unable to entertain a complex three column formulation or even a simple reframing of her difficulties as part of a broader pattern of interaction that included the family and involved professionals. In Positive Practice it is recognized that parents need a chance to ventilate overwhelming emotions, often by discussing simplistic black and white descriptions of the problem and simplified solutions like hospitalization or reception into care. The expression of empathy for the overwhelming feelings with which parents are faced is therefore important. However, this empathy and support must be given without accepting the simplistic problem definitions and solutions that accompany the intense emotions. Here are some typical examples of constructive empathy and contrasting examples of collusion in black and white thinking and individualistic problem formulations and solutions. This is constructive empathy.

- *It sounds like you're really worried about her. You're driven to distraction wondering what she will do next.*
- *You have both been in a battle and now she has walked out. This has left you with a deep feeling of loss and failure.*

This is destructive collusion

- *It sounds like you see her as really agitated and needing something to calm her down. Well, I will phone the GP and ask that he consider medication.*
- *You see her running away as a sign of delinquency and you see boarding school as a way of containing that. I can suggest two places you could call.*

It is not intended in these examples to give the impression that medication and residential placement have no place in Positive Practice. Far from it. Many excellent examples of how these interventions may be integrated into systemic approaches to formulating and resolving a variety of very difficult problems have been described (e.g. Falloon et al, 1993; Manor, 1991). Rather, the central point is that it is not Positive Practice to use these interventions within the context of a formulation that labels one system member as *bad, sad, sick* or mad and the other members of the system as being uninvolved in the maintenance or resolution of the problem.

3. Acknowledge that labelling one person as the problem would provide short term relief but may lead to long term difficulties

Defining complex interactional problems in simple individual terms usually provides short term relief for parents. Individual problem definitions (like *sad, bad, sick* or *mad*) usually entail clear unambiguous solutions. These allow parents a way of avoiding the emotional pain which goes with exploring an interactional problem formulation and carrying out the solutions that follow from it. However, in the long term simplistic solutions to individual framings of interactional problems may lead to major difficulties.

For example, when children are defined as *sad* or depressed, the simplistic solution is to cheer them up by arranging for them to join the scouts, go to a sports club or take up a hobby to make them happy. In the long term, the child may find that scouts, sports and hobbies leave them as sad as ever. Both the parents and the child may be left with a sense of despair that the depression is unresolvable, and anger that the solution did not work.

Punishment is the simplistic solution for *bad* or delinquent children. In the long run, sustained punishment untempered by understanding and warmth leads children to become alienated from their parents. This alienation may lead to further conduct problems. Punishment may take many forms from physical or verbal abuse to threats of abandonment or actual placement of the child in care or a boarding school situation. That is not to say that residential and foster care or boarding schools are necessarily alienating or destructive. Rather, the point is, that if the child sees the placement as an act of punishment, then it may lead to alienation and this may further compound the problem.

Hospitalization, individual assessment or therapy and medication are the more common simple solutions suggested when youngsters are defined as *mad, sick,* or mentally ill. All three of these interventions, when used outside of an interactional systemic framing of the problem, run the risk of confirming the youngster's identity as a problem person, victim, or invalid. Once youngsters accept this type of problem-saturated identity, their problem behaviour may increase and the quality of their relationships with their parents may deteriorate.

In my clinical experience no parents want to reap the potentially disastrous consequences that may arise from individualistic framings of their children's problems. They do not want to run the risk of casting their children into despair, destruction, alienation or invalidity. However, they are often unaware that individualistic framings have these long term consequences. An important part of crisis management in Positive Practice is to acknowledge parent's understandable wish to avoid the emotional pain that pushes parents to adopt individualistic framings of the problem, and to point out to them the destructive long-term consequences that may inadvertently arise from their individualistic construction of their children's problem behaviour.

4. Offer an urgent appointment and a plan

When a crisis occurs, parents may feel helpless and threatened yet aware that they must take action. Once they have ventilated their feelings and seen that individualistic problem definitions and simplistic solutions are inappropriate, they will feel supported. However, they may still be at a loss to know how to proceed. In Positive Practice, it is crucial to help parents form an immediate action plan. It has already been mentioned that this plan should offer precedence to managing risks of danger. A second priority is that it will maximize the chances of them accepting the interactional problem formulation and related solutions.

A useful place to start constructing such a plan is to decide on a date for the next appointment. This should be as soon as possible. During crises, people are open to accepting new framings of old problems. Usually, the further from a crises a family moves, the less open it will be to change. A second consideration is who should attend the post-crisis consultation. In Positive Practice, significant members of the wider network, including involved professionals and important members of the extended family, may be included in the consultation. With the Barrows, Caroline's year-head, the GP and the school nurse were invited to the post-crisis consultation. Where important members of the network are unavailable for this consultation, the therapist may phone them beforehand, inform them of the situation, request comments and relay this information to those who attend the consultation. These absent network members should be briefed after the consultation as to the outcome and about the plan.

Once a decision has been reached on the time, place and composition of the post-crisis consultation, the parents or children may be offered a plan to carry out between the phonecall and the consultation. Often the most appropriate plan is to monitor a specific aspect of the situation or to avoid engaging in escalating patterns of behaviour. With Caroline, she talked explicitly to me about the importance of being left alone in her room and asked that her parents respect her right to do this during the forty-eight hour period before the post-crisis consultation. Here are some examples of tasks given to family members during crisis phonecalls.

- *Between now and the meeting tomorrow, there are a couple of things that you can do that may provide useful information for yourself and your family. First, notice those situations where the sense of tension in the house subsides and keep a note of the time and circumstances surrounding these episodes. Second, if you feel yourself being drawn into a typical bickering session, tell Marie that you have been asked by me to avoid this until after tomorrow's meeting and then make a cup of tea instead of continuing.*

- *We will meet in three days. Tonight, tomorrow night and Thursday night may be stressful for you. You may want to know what is the best thing to do. May I suggest this? Follow your usual routine of putting the kids to bed, doing the story and then watching the news. But after that, phone Colin and tell him in detail about how you managed the strong feelings of anger that you felt during the routine. Rate these on a ten point scale. We can discuss the fluctuations in your feelings at the meeting on Friday.*
- *You may find that the urge to run away becomes very strong. If you don't know what to do, here is something that another boy in your sort of situation found useful. He would lock himself in his room and then write a letter to me telling me why he had to run away and why he found it difficult to do so. You may find this sort of thing useful. If you do decide to write me some letters, we can set aside time on Monday for you and I to read them privately. Or you may wish to keep them a secret. Its up to you. But the thing is, the writing itself may help you contain the urge to run away.*

A list of the guidelines for managing crises is presented in Figure 13.5.

GUIDELINES FOR MANAGING A CRISIS PHONECALL

1. Assess and manage danger
2. Empathize with the caller's emotional pain without colluding with their simplistic solutions
3. Acknowledge that labelling one person as the problem would provide short term relief but may lead to long term difficulties
4. Offer an urgent appointment and a plan
5. Significant network members should be included in the post-crisis consultation
6. The plan for managing the situation until the post-crisis consultation should include symptom monitoring tasks and tasks that prevent the escalation of destructive interactional spirals

---

Figure 13.5.   Crisis phonecalls

SUMMARY

A therapeutic dilemma is a concise statement of the disadvantages and difficulties associated with leaving the presenting problem unresolved and the disadvantages and risks entailed by solving the problem. If clients see that they have not got the personal resources to cope with the demands of either living with the problem or taking steps towards its resolution, stating the therapeutic dilemma may precipitate a therapeutic crisis. Invariably, therapeutic crises involve some family members doubting the interactional three column formulation of the problem and redefining the problem as an individual difficulty rather than as an interactional phenomenon. That is, someone in the family becomes defined as *bad, sad, sick* or *mad*. The pressure to collude with the family and other network members in abandoning an interactional construction of the problem and accepting an individual description is usually very intense.

In Positive Practice, the following guidelines for handling crisis phonecalls help therapists avoid this collusive process. First, assess and manage the risk of danger, self-injury or abuse. Second, empathize with the caller's emotional pain without colluding with their simplistic solutions. Third, acknowledge that labelling one person as the problem would provide short term relief but may lead to long term difficulties. Fourth, offer an urgent appointment and a plan. Significant network members should be included in the post-crisis consultation. The plan for managing the situation until the post-crisis consultation should include symptom monitoring tasks and tasks that prevent the escalation of destructive interactional spirals.

The importance of a crisis is that it presents the family with a severe problem to manage. Fortunately, the more severe a problem is, the greater the motivation of the clients to co-operate with a therapist provided they view the therapist as competent to help them. Families are more likely to view therapists as competent if they follow the crisis phonecall management guidelines described in this chapter.

Exercise 13.1.

Select a family that one member of the training group is currently seeing, that has recently been involved in a therapeutic crisis.

This member, in conjunction with the group must summarize the case by drawing a genogram and a three column formulation.

Divide the training group into members who will role-play the family, and members who will act as therapist and team.

Family members should take about 10 minutes talking together agreeing in detail about how the crisis occurred and how they feel about it.

The therapist must then conduct a 10 minute one-to-one interview with the concerned family member as if it were a crisis phonecall. Follow the guidelines for managing crisis phonecalls set out in Figure 13.5.

Derole after the exercise.

Take 20 minutes to discuss
1.   The experience of the concerned family member who participated in the crisis one-to-one interview
2.   The areas in which the therapist felt competent and the areas in which the therapist felt challenged when managing the one-to-one interview.

Exercise 13. 2. Outline.

You have been working with the White family for 5 sessions while Karen was on an inpatient behavioural weight gain programme on the paediatrics ward of a general hospital. You sent the letter set out below to recap the pre-discharge session and the contract for further work. The work so far has helped you to construct the three column formulation outlined below. You also know that Karen is the only child in this relatively isolated family. Karen achieved her target weight during the programme and was discharged a week ago. Karen has maintained this weight since discharge. However, she is now openly defying her parents and demanding more autonomy and privacy. She is arguing about these issues rather than food and dieting. The father, Tom, calls to your office alone and demands Karen be hospitalized and sedated because Karen threw a tantrum and then locked herself in her room after they reprimanded her for staying out late. He insists that she is seriously disturbed and requires individual therapy only.

Divide the training group into members who will role-play the family and members who will act as therapist and team.

Family members should take about 10 minutes talking together agreeing in detail about how the crisis occurred and how they feel about it.

The therapist must then conduct a 10 minute one-to-one interview with John White (the father) as if it were a crisis phonecall. Follow the guidelines for managing crisis phonecalls set out in Figure 13.5.

Derole after the exercise.

Take 20 minutes to discuss
1.   The experience of John in the crisis one-to-one interview
2.   The areas in which the therapist felt competent and the areas in which the therapist felt challenged when managing the one-to-one interview.

Child and Family Clinic
Market Town
Norfolk

2.5.90

Mr and Mrs White
15 Broad Street
Market Town

Dear John and Barbara

We covered a lot of ground in a very stormy and stressful session today before Karen was discharged. This is a note just to recap the main points. No-one can say with any certainty what caused your daughters anorexia. Today we did, however, make a formulation that explains why it persists. A copy of the formulation is appended to this letter. Karen is clearly trapped with you in a cycle of interaction that is very upsetting for all of you. We are confident, however, that each of you has the personal strength to break out of this cycle and prevent Karen's starvation. We suggest the following three point plan to help you with this.

First, once her weight is out of the danger zone we advise that she take responsibility for keeping her weight within normal limits. In practice this means that you will no longer have to remind her to eat sensibly. Her weight and her eating habits will be her own business.

Second, as soon as Karen can show that she is capable of maintaining her body weight outside the danger zone for six consecutive months we will no longer need to monitor her. She may choose to have her weight checked regularly here or at your family doctor's surgery. If her weight falls into the danger zone she will immediately be readmitted to an inpatient weight gain programme.

Third, you need to encourage Karen to negotiate for the degree of privacy and autonomy that is typical for a fourteen year old. At present she settles for the level of privacy and autonomy that is appropriate for a nine year old girl, not a fourteen year old teenager. She seems to put all her energy into arguing with you both about food instead of negotiating about growing up. We are happy to facilitate this negotiation process and suggest that you meet with us for a series of six one-hour consultations to focus on this.

As we said to you today, if you are able to commit yourselves to following through on all three aspects of this plan then there is an excellent chance that the starvation process can be reversed.

We look forward to seeing you again on Thursday May 12th at 2.00pm.

Yours sincerely

Dr Alan Carr

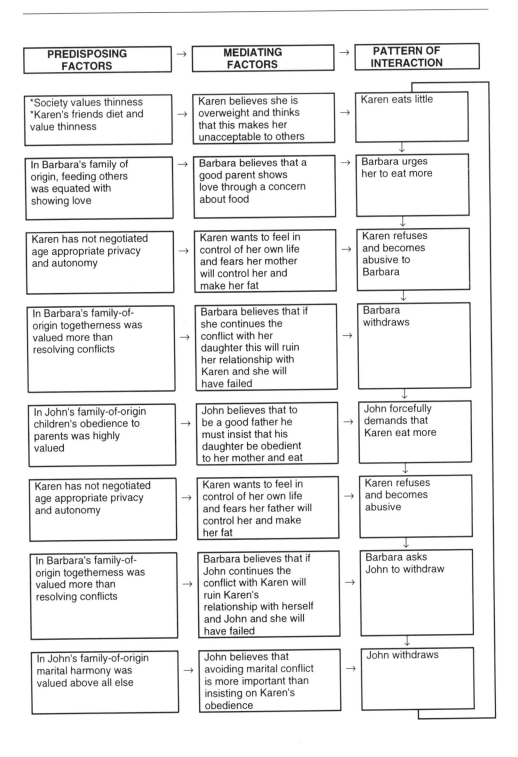

PREDISPOSING FACTORS	→	MEDIATING FACTORS	→	PATTERN OF INTERACTION
*Society values thinness *Karen's friends diet and value thinness	→	Karen believes she is overweight and thinks that this makes her unacceptable to others	→	Karen eats little
In Barbara's family of origin, feeding others was equated with showing love	→	Barbara believes that a good parent shows love through a concern about food	→	Barbara urges her to eat more
Karen has not negotiated age appropriate privacy and autonomy	→	Karen wants to feel in control of her own life and fears her mother will control her and make her fat	→	Karen refuses and becomes abusive to Barbara
In Barbara's family-of-origin togetherness was valued more than resolving conflicts	→	Barbara believes that if she continues the conflict with her daughter this will ruin her relationship with Karen and she will have failed	→	Barbara withdraws
In John's family-of-origin children's obedience to parents was highly valued	→	John believes that to be a good father he must insist that his daughter be obedient to her mother and eat	→	John forcefully demands that Karen eat more
Karen has not negotiated age appropriate privacy and autonomy	→	Karen wants to feel in control of her own life and fears her father will control her and make her fat	→	Karen refuses and becomes abusive
In Barbara's family-of-origin togetherness was valued more than resolving conflicts	→	Barbara believes that if John continues the conflict with Karen will ruin Karen's relationship with herself and John and she will have failed	→	Barbara asks John to withdraw
In John's family-of-origin marital harmony was valued above all else	→	John believes that avoiding marital conflict is more important than insisting on Karen's obedience	→	John withdraws

Exercise 13.2.   Three column formulation for the White family

14

Individual Consultations and Talking to Children

With the Barrow case a network meeting was held two days after the crisis phonecall. The following people attended: Dick, Sheila and Caroline Barrow; the GP, Dr Wilson; the school nurse, Sarah Boyd; the Education and Welfare Officer, Phil Hutchinson and the year-head Ms Hackett. This was the fifth consultation.

Prior to the network meeting I met with Caroline alone for an individual interview. In this chapter a description of this consultation will be given, along with some guidelines for managing individual consultations with children as part of a broader programme of systemic consultation. Consideration will also be given to specific techniques for including children in the family therapy process generally.

THE INDIVIDUAL CONSULTATION WITH CAROLINE

An individual consultation with Caroline was conducted prior to the network meeting for a number of reasons. The first reason for seeing Caroline alone, was to assess suicidal intent. The possibility of self-harm had been raised by Dick during the crisis phonecall. My hunch was that this was unlikely, given that Caroline had denied any suicidal ideation during the crisis telephone call. Nevertheless, it was important to check this again.

The second reason for seeing Caroline alone was to clarify her view of her current situation. I believed that Caroline would find it less threatening to tell me her view in private than in a large network meeting. In Positive Practice when a team is managing a case, a specific team member can be assigned to form a relationship with a youngster and to act as an advocate in wider network meetings. In the individual session with Caroline, I opened up the possibility of acting as her advocate within the overall network meeting. However, it was important to distinguish the role of advocate from that of consultant to the overall system. I made this distinction with Caroline and later with the members of the system in the network consultation. This was done to preserve a position of neutrality within the overall therapeutic system.

The third reason for seeing Caroline alone was because I guessed that Dick's insistence that Caroline required individual treatment for a personal psychological disturbance would prevent the members of the network from exploring other possibilities. If I could inform the meeting that I had evaluated Caroline's psychological state prior to the meeting and found her to be understandably upset but not seriously disturbed, then the meeting would not be constrained by an individualistic framing of the problem.

The atmosphere of the meeting with Caroline was fairly relaxed and informal. She and I shared a particular interest in Terry Prachett's Discworld comic-fantasy novels. The Discworld is flat and travels through the universe on the back of a Giant Turtle. Many people on Discworld do not believe this. Rather, they believe that the world is round and come to grief when they try to circumnavigate it. They sail off the edge into the abyss. Caroline said she that felt like one of the people on Discworld who tried to warn sailors of the dangers of attempting circumnavigation. No one took her seriously when she described her abdominal pains. The pains were getting worse. She rated them at eight on a ten point scale. She was angry at both of her parents for ganging up on her and just wanted to be left to get on with her life alone. She wished that she could be given space like her brother Mat to be herself. She worried about her mother, Sheila and she wished that her father, Dick was more regularly available to support Sheila. She still felt disbelieved by the GP, Dr Wilson, and was angry that he accused her of malingering.

Looking to the future, she said that she would go to school and put up with the pains if everyone would just leave her alone.

Her mood was low but she expressed no suicidal ideation or intention.

She said that she would like me to represent her position, as summarized here, in the network meeting but did not want the extent of her anger towards the GP, Dr Wilson, mentioned. I agreed to this.

Immediately following this individual session, the network meeting was convened. This will be described in the next chapter. Now let us turn to the general problem of including children in family therapy and to broad guidelines for conducting individual child centred consultations as part of family therapy.

FITTING INDIVIDUAL SESSIONS INTO THE SYSTEMIC CONSULTATION PROCESS

There was a time in the evolution of family therapy when the effects of concurrent individual and family consultations were thought to be antagonistic rather than synergistic (e.g., Haley, 1980; Selvini Palazzoli and Prata, 1982). This belief was not without foundation. In some cases, when one family member receives individual work it confirms an individualistic problem framing and works against the family accepting a broader interactional formulation of the presenting problem. This usually occurs where the formulation is unclear, where the objective of the individual consultations is unclear and where the roles of team members have not been clearly negotiated.

For example, a trainee psychologist was assigned to conduct unspecified *individual work* with a nine year old boy who was referred because of reading difficulties and aggressive school based problems. The supervisor, who adopted the role of the systems consultant, met with the child, the trainee and the parents periodically. Within these meetings the trainee felt unsure about how to describe the focus of the individual work with the child or how to indicate to what extent progress was being made, because no overall formulation had been co-constructed by the supervisor, the trainee and the family. Within the family sessions, attempts by the supervisor to help the parents develop a plan for cooperating with the school in dealing with the child's difficulties were repeatedly thwarted. The parents would highlight the fact that the child liked the individual sessions and needed more of these to get better.

Not all cases of concurrent individual and family consultation need flounder like this one. The assessment value or therapeutic impact of concurrent individual and family sessions may be synergistic or complimentary provided certain conditions are met (Carr and Afnan, 1989; Carr, Gawlinski et al, 1989; Carr, McDonnell et al, 1989). First, individual consultations must be planned within a systemic context. Second, there should be a clear set of objectives for individual consultations. Third, the way of working within the consultation should clearly address the objectives of the consultations. Fourth, there should be agreement on the limits of confidentiality and the degree to which information from the individual consultations may be shared and the way in which this is fed back into family meetings. Fifth, the roles of child advocate or key worker and consultant to the family and wider system must be clearly differentiated, particularly when one worker fulfils both roles. Where individual consultations and family consultations are conducted by separate team members, the way in which these team members work together must be clearly negotiated.

FUNCTIONS OF INDIVIDUAL SESSIONS

Individual sessions may be used to fulfil different functions at different stages in the consultation process (Carr, 1994b). During the assessment phase of consultation before a systemic formulation has been elaborated, individual sessions may fruitfully be used to establish the young person's view of the problem, the pattern of interaction around it, and the beliefs which they hold that trap them in this pattern. A child-centred assessment session plan for use in Positive Practice will be given below. During the assessment phase, individual sessions are also useful for establishing youngsters' abilities and achievements, particularly if attainment problems have been reported or are suspected. In this context, it is worth mentioning that conduct problems are by far the commonest presenting problem in child and family clinics, and there is a well established association between conduct problems and academic difficulties (Kazdin, 1991).

Once a systemic formulation has been co-constructed, individual sessions may be used to help youngsters develop skills to break out of the pattern of interaction around the presenting problem. Training programmes that help youngsters develop communication skills, problem solving skills, self control strategies, study skills and social skills have been particularly well developed within the cognitive behavioural tradition. Kratochwill and Morris' (1991) text is a useful starting point for finding treatment manuals which describe these programmes. Within Positive Practice, children may also use individual sessions once a systemic formulation has been co-constructed to evolve new belief systems, belief systems which will help them to avoid repeating the behaviour which keeps them trapped in the pattern of interaction around the presenting problem. Play therapies which have developed within the client-centred and psycho-analytic traditions and the more recent integrative approaches offer fruitful avenues for helping children evolve new belief systems. A good account of the major schools of play therapy is given in Schaefer and O'Connor's (1993) handbook. O'Connor's (1991) own integrative approach is well described in a useful treatment manual.

At any point in the systemic consultation process where a crisis occurs, individual sessions help clinician's assess the risk of youngsters being in danger of abuse, suicide or violence directed towards others. The process of dealing with children who say that they have been abused or are at risk of abuse is complex, especially when the abuse is sexual. A useful guide for interviewing children in such circumstances is Jones and McQuiston's (1988) *Interviewing the Sexually Abused Child*. The assessment of suicide risk is a crucial skill for crisis management in Positive Practice and guidelines for this will be given below. Guidance on the individual assessment of dangerousness is difficult to give because of the conflicting evidence on this issue (see for example DeKraai and Sales, 1991). The single certainty in this area is that a history of previous violent episodes is predictive of future violent episodes (Macrae, 1978).

INDIVIDUAL SESSION ASSESSMENT PLAN

An individual assessment plan for use with children in Positive Practice is summarized in Figure 14.1. The following example illustrates the way in which the assessment plan may be used in practice.

Derek and Maureen Dineen came with their son Finbar, aged nine, for a private consultation. They were worried about the increasing conflict between Maureen and Finbar. Sometimes their arguments became so heated that Maureen felt she would lose control and injure Finbar. After a preliminary family interview, it was clear that the cycle of interaction around the problem often began when Maureen attended to Finbar's youngest sister Gail. Then, he would act in a way that led to a reprimand from Maureen. This in turn would lead to a rapid-fire symmetrical escalation of negative comments between mother and son. It would end with Maureen putting Finbar in the coal shed for a period. He would then come out and the incident would apparently be closed.

Both parents were certain that there was something deeply psychologically wrong with Finbar and believed that an individual assessment of their son was vital. Further-more, a previous psychological assessment of Finbar had shown that his IQ fell within the superior range of abilities and that he was therefore a *gifted child*. Maureen and Derek wondered if this contributed to the family's problems. It was also difficult to understand Finbar's position because he said little during the family interview and sat cowering in the corner.

1. Clarify expectations

The individual session was carried out a week after the intake interview. In the first minutes of the session I explained to Finbar what he could expect. Here are some of the things I said to clarify the agenda.

```
┌─────────────────────────────────────────────────────────────────────┐
│                                                                       │
│                        CHILD CENTRED SESSION                          │
│                                                                       │
│        1. Clarify what the child may expect                           │
│                    Session duration                                   │
│                    Purpose of session                                 │
│                    The child's right to privacy                       │
│                                                                       │
│        2. Describe other's views of the problem                       │
│                    Parents                                            │
│                    Teachers                                           │
│                    Involved professionals                             │
│                                                                       │
│        3. Clarify the child's view of the problem                     │
│                    The exact difficulties                             │
│                    The pattern of interaction around it               │
│                    The child's attempted solutions                    │
│                                                                       │
│        4. Clarify the child's view of the family                      │
│                    Genogram                                           │
│                    Lifeline                                           │
│                    Emotions                                           │
│                                                                       │
│        5. Clarify the child's view of the future                      │
│                    Picture of the present                             │
│                    Picture of the future                              │
│                                                                       │
│        6. Formulate and summarize                                     │
│                                                                       │
│        7. Agree on feedback                                           │
│                                                                       │
└─────────────────────────────────────────────────────────────────────┘
```

Figure 14.1.   Child-centred assessment checklist

Duration of the session:
- *This session will last about an hour: about the same length of time as Sesame Street. Then you and your mum will drive home. OK?*

Purpose of the session:
- *I want to talk to you because I want to help yourself and your Mum find a way to stop fighting so much. I know that the fighting probably makes you sad. So maybe today we can talk about escaping.......escaping and getting away from that sadness.*

Child's right to privacy:
- *There are no right or wrong answers to any of the questions that I ask you. So you can just tell me what you believe. But only talk to me about things you want to talk about.*
- *Your mum and dad need to understand your side of the story. So when we have finished talking today, we can both decide how to explain it to them. There may be some things that you really want them to know about. There may be others that you want to keep private. That's OK.*

This last area is an ethically challenging one. It is your duty to protect children in potentially dangerous situations. So, if a child talks about abuse or potentially abusive situations, then you have a duty to act to protect the child. Indeed in countries where legislation has been passed requiring the mandatory reporting of cases of child abuse, a professional may break the law by not acting when children say that they have been abused. On the other hand, if you tell a child that you will not respect his or her desire for privacy and confidentiality if there is a danger of abuse, you may rule out the possibility of developing a trusting relationship with the child and obtaining an accurate understanding of their world view. This dilemma is an ethical challenge for all of us who conduct child centred assessments. This and related issues will be discussed more fully in Chapter 17.

2. Tell the child what others think about the problem

In Finbar's case, it was important that he understand his parent's view of the problem and their wish to resolve it. Here is one of the ways this was expressed so that he could make sense of how his mother felt.

- *Last week, Finbar, your mum was saying how well the two of you got along together until about two years ago. She said the two of you used to curl up in the armchair together in front of the fire and watch TV. That doesn't happen any more. She would like to be able to do that again. But she doesn't know how to. So that is her view of the problem.*

Part of the therapist's job in an individual session is to frame the view of significant members of the child's network to the child in a way that is intelligible to the child and in a way that helps the child construe their relationship with other members of the network in as positive or useful a way as possible. In the case of Finbar, I did not frame his mother's position as *she wants you to stop being naughty* because this individualistic negative framing would not open up possibilities of forming a more positive relationship with his mother. Rather I chose to frame the mother's position as one of sadness about losing her close positive relationship with Finbar: a relationship she wanted to regain. This relational positive framing opened up possibilities for Finbar exploring how he might contribute to this quest.

In complex cases, teachers, foster parents, social workers, family doctors and so forth may each hold different views of the problem. Framing these views intelligibly and positively for the child so that he or she may respond to the various positions of significant network members is an important part of the child centred consultation.

3. Clarify the child's view of the problem

When the child is clear on what to expect during the session and on the views of significant members of her network, then the therapist may move on to making space for the child to present their view of the problem. In Positive Practice the plan for assessing the child's view of the problem within the context of an individual session is conceptually similar to the plan for conducting a family assessment with a view to constructing a three column formulation. That is, first the child's description of the pattern of interaction around the presenting problem is clarified. Then, the child's view of the beliefs that trap family members into this cycle is brought forth. In particular, the child's beliefs about the nature of the problem and the types of strategies that may be used to solve it are discussed. Many of the interviewing strategies discussed in Chapters 5 and 6 may be used with older children and adolescents.

With young children, techniques which capitalize upon the child's interest in play materials and concrete thinking style are often far more productive than straight interviewing. Dolls, puppets and drawings may be used to help children define problems and track sequences of interaction around the problems in a theatrical way.

In Finbar's case, I suggested that we start the session by doing some drawings. He spontaneously drew a cartoon sequence involving Bart Simpson and himself. I suggested that he draw a cartoon sequence to illustrate what happens when he and his mother argue. I asked that each window of the cartoon be put on a separate page. This allowed me to ask him to clarify what happened between windows and to draw new pictures to fill in gaps in the sequence. He began with only three windows. In the first, his mother shouted at him to pick up his coat. In the second, he shouted *NO!!* In the third, he was in the coal shed. When we completed this part of the assessment, his cartoon had seven windows as follows: The first began with him feeling annoyed when he saw his mother fussing over the baby because he believed that she saw the baby as a replacement for him. The second showed a picture of him pretending to be an angel and his mother ignoring him. The third showed him being a devil and throwing his coat on the floor in temper. The fourth showed his mother reprimanding him. The fifth showed him shouting *NO!!* In the sixth frame he was in the coal shed. The sequence ended with him slipping out of the door under a rain cloud, while his parents, sister and the baby were all together watching television. This expanded sequence was elicited by asking:

- *What's going on between here and here? (while pointing to two cartoon frames).*

The same question may fruitfully be used with younger children who are dramatizing a sequence using dolls and a dolls house or puppets.

4. Clarify the child's view of the family

By clarifying the child's view of the family, a backdrop is provided against which to flesh out with the child possible beliefs of other family members that constrain them in the pattern of interaction around the problem.

In Chapter 6, we looked at the use of genograms and developmental histories as general assessment methods. Both of these assessment methods may be used in individual consultations with children to construct their view of the family. Both procedures may be presented as games. Drawing a genogram is a game the object of which is to draw a map of everyone in the family. The rules are that squares are for boys and circles for girls. Every circle or square must have a name and an age in it. And so on. When the basic genogram is finished, more detailed information about the child's perception of family members and family patterns may be included (McGoldrick and Gerson, 1985).

A developmental family history can be represented pictorially on the whiteboard as a family lifeline. Significant events in the development of the family, such as births, deaths, starting school, changing house, and so on, may be included on the lifeline to furnish a spatial representation of the family's evolution over time.

Once a genogram and lifeline are drawn, the child's perception of emotional aspects of family life may be brought forth as follows. First, draw faces representing four basic emotions, as set out in Figure 14.2, beside the genogram and ask what emotions they represent. Then ask the following sorts of questions to establish how the child views the current and past emotional climate within the family.

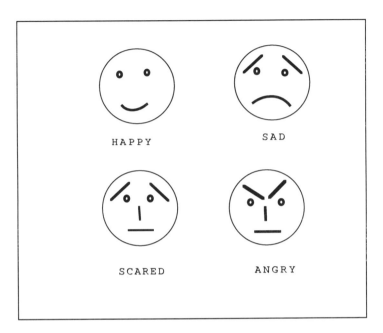

Figure 14.2.   Faces to use when asking children about the emotional climate of the family

- *Who in the genogram is most sad/happy/scared/angry at the moment?*
- *Who is least sad/happy/scared/angry?*

Help the child to draw the faces representing the emotion beside the person feeling it on the genogram. Then probe why the family members feel these emotions. Here are some typical problems:

- *What happened to make Mummy/Daddy/Mary feel so sad/happy/scared/angry?*
- *What did he/she think when that was happening?*

Move on to explore changes in the emotional climate of the family over time.

- *Do you see this point on the lifeline? Who was most/least sad/happy/scared/angry then?*

Then follow these types of questions up with probes about what happened to make people feel as they did, and what they believed about the events that led to their emotional states.

Finbar's genogram and lifeline are contained in Figures 14.3 and 14.4. From these it is was clear that Finbar felt that himself and his father were sad because they were excluded from a relationship with Maureen since the birth of Gail. The difficulties associated with this seemed to lead Maeve, his six year old sister, to be worried or scared. He loved school from the day he started and all of the difficulties seemed to be home based.

5. Clarify the child's view of the future

In Chapter 8, goal setting with families was explored. The principles of goal setting described in Chapter 8 may be applied to individual consultations with children. A

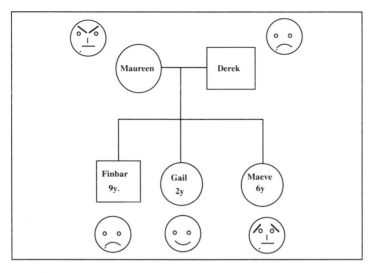

Figure 14.3. Finbar's genogram

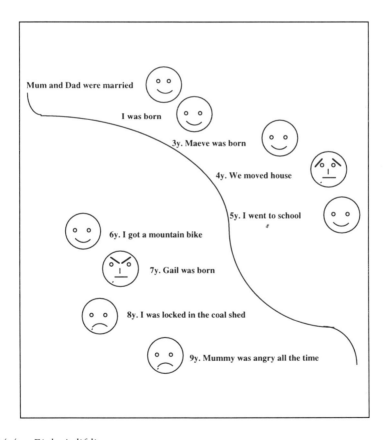

Figure 14.4. Finbar's lifeline

particularly engaging way to help children describe their goals in concrete terms is to ask them to draw a picture of the family as it would be in six months time if everything worked out right for them. Then, interview them about what each person in the family is thinking, feeling and doing.

A variation on this technique is to ask children to draw a picture of their family as it is now and as it would be in six months' time if everything turned out right and then ask them to highlight the differences between the two pictures. In particular how are the beliefs, feelings and actions of family members were different.

With the Dineen case, Finbar's picture of the future portrayed him sitting beside his mum on the couch with Derek holding Gail, and Maeve sitting on the floor. All family members were watching television and laughing. The coal shed had been converted into a playroom and there was a Nintendo computer in there that Finbar could use whenever he liked.

6. Summarize the child's view and agree on feedback

At the conclusion of a child centred consultation, the therapist pulls together the child's view of the problem, the pattern of interaction in which it is embedded, the family and the future into a three column formulation, albeit a simplified formulation relying only on the child's account. Finbar's view of his situation was summarized into the three column formulation set out in Figure 14.5. I talked him through it and he said that he could see clearly how *the pieces of the jigsaw puzzle fit together.* I then linked the formulation to his goals by noting that he wanted to arrive at a situation where he could be friends with his mum and where the fights would not occur as often but that he did not know how to get there. He agreed to have the summary presented in full to his parents at the next family session. That family session was particularly moving. When Maureen saw Finbar's view of the situation set out in detail, she found herself able to empathize with her son. The angry stand-off that she and Finbar had been stuck in began to dissolve. The similarity between Derek and Finbar's emotional positions was also a focus for therapy which aimed at strengthening the father-son relationship. With increased empathy between Maureen and Finbar and a closer bond between Finbar and Derek, Finbar found that he was less likely to interpret his mother's positive interactions with Gail as a rejection of himself.

SUICIDE AND INDIVIDUAL CONSULTATIONS

Suicide is not a rare event. For example in Ireland, one person commits suicide every day (Clarke-Finnegan and Fahy, 1983). When crises occur and youngsters mention self-harm, an individual consultation is an important adjunct to a family consultation. The threat of self-harm is most usefully construed as a youngster's attempt to solve a dilemma that he or she faces. It is useful to think of it as a solution to a major problem which probably involves significant members of the family and wider social network. In some instances, youngsters actually intend to end their lives. In others, the threat of self-harm is used as a way of indicating to the family or members of their network that the youngster has a serious problem with which he or she cannot cope and for which help is

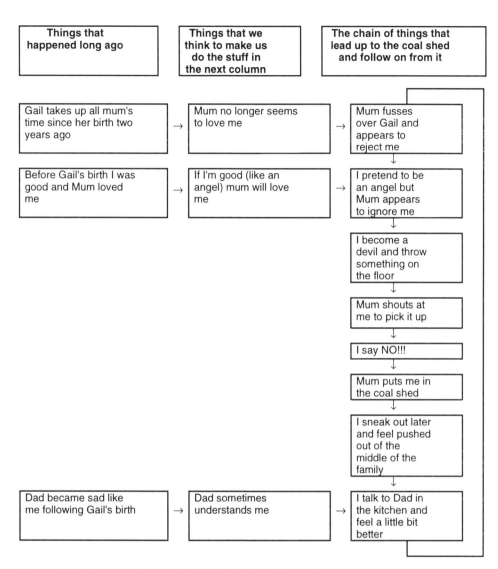

Figure 14.5. Summary formulation of Finbar's view of the problem

required. These two different scenarios are referred to as suicide and parasuicide respectively (Hawton, 1992).

In Positive Practice, with cases where there is a risk of self harm, the therapist's task is to engage with clients in co-constructing a three column formulation, with self-injurious thoughts, feelings or actions as the central problem. It is fruitful to conduct this type of consultation from an informed position. Extensive empirical research on both suicide and parasuicide has furnished us with lists of risk factors associated with suicide and parasuicide. These are summarized in Figure 14.7. This list and the following discussion are based on comprehensive surveys of the empirical literature contained in Berman and Jobes, 1993; Orbach, 1988; Hawton, 1992 and Hawton and

Catalan, 1982. Obviously only some of the risk factors in Figure 14.7 are relevant to children or adolescents. However, the full list is included, since in some cases parents present with problems related to self-harm. The risk factors have been clustered in such a way so that inquiries about them may be easily included in a systemic consultation to cases where there is a risk of self harm. Like all empirically identified risk factors, the presence of a number of them alerts the therapist to the increased probability that the phenomenon in question may occur in a particular clinical case. Before detailing a method for conducting an individual consultation with a child or adolescent in a case where self-harm is at issue, let me place such individual consultation procedures within the context of a global systemic assessment.

The overriding objective of a family consultation where self-harm has been threatened is to prevent harm, injury or death from occurring.

Certain broad principles for assessment may be followed. First, if there is an immediate risk of self-harm, offer immediate consultation. Second, use the consultation process to co-construct the most useful possible understanding of the situation surrounding the threat of self-harm. Third, during the consultation process, establish or deepen your working alliance with all significant members of the network. Fourth, in coconstructing a three column formulation of the self- injurious thoughts feelings and actions, make inquires and observations related to all relevant risk factors in Figure 14.7. Check if the factors were present in the past, the extent to which they were present during the recent episode, and whether they are immediately present. Where possible obtain information relating to risk factors from as many members of the network as possible. This includes the youngster who has threatened self-harm, key members of the family, and previously involved professionals. Fifth, identify people within the youngster's social network and the network of involved professionals that may contribute to the solution of the presenting problems. Sixth, draw the information you obtain into a clear formulation on which a management plan can be based. The formulation must logically link the risk factors identified in the case together to explain the occurrence of the episode of self-injurious behaviour and the current level of risk. It is useful, in addition to the three column formulation, to specify the *precipitating factors* that immediately preceded the pattern of interaction around the self-injurious features to escalate from ideation to intention or from intention to action. The management plan must specify the short term action to be taken in the light of the formulation. The plan must logically indicate that the changes it entails will probably lower the risk of self-harm.

The following guidelines provide a framework for conducting an individual assessment in cases of self-harm. Usually this consultation will follow a family interview, so you will have the parents' and other involved professionals' accounts of how the concern about self-harm occurred.

1. Clarify expectations and the limits of confidentiality

As with the routine child-centred assessment interview described earlier in this chapter, it is important first to let the child know the duration of the interview and what will follow on from it. If hospitalization or some other protective intervention is an option, it is better to mention that it is a possible outcome than to conceal it.

RISK FACTOR CATEGORIES	FACTORS ASSOCIATED WITH SUICIDE RISK	CORRELATES OF REPEATED PARASUICIDE
Suicidal intent	Advanced planning Precautions to avoid discovery No attempt to gain help afterwards Dangerous method Final act	Suicidal ideation without intent
Immediate circumstances	Sequence of events leading to hopelessness,	Impulsive separation following relationship difficulties Family illness Recent court appearance
Network characteristics	Recent stressful life events and losses Denial by family of seriousness of intent Child abuse or spouse abuse Social isolation Recent unemployment	Social isolation through social mobility Crowding Chronic unemployment
Psychological history	Previous suicide attempt Depression Antisocial personality disorder Alcohol and drug abuse	Previous suicide attempt Dysthymia Loss of parent in early life Antisocial personality disorder Criminal record Alcohol and drug abuse Previous psychiatric treatment
Medical history	Chronic painful physical illness Epilepsy	Epilepsy
Demographic profile and seasonal factors	Male Young (18-25) or old (over 50) Divorced, marital discord or widowed SES group 1 or 5 Season: early summer	Female Teenager or Young Adult Single, teenage wife, divorced SES group 5

Figure 14.6. Risk factors in suicide and parasuicide

It is also crucial to be accurate about the limits of confidentiality. You must let the child know that you will not break a confidence that they ask you to keep unless it is necessary for keeping them safe.

You cannot move into the heart of the consultation until you have joined with the youngster and established rapport. It may be useful to start by inquiring about some relatively unthreatening area like schoolwork or friendships. Once you have joined with the youngster, move into the central part of the interview.

2. Explore suicidal ideation, suicidal intention and self-injurious behaviour

In cases where a suicide attempt has been made, obtain a detailed description of the self-destructive behaviour that led to the referral and all related suicidal ideation and intentions. Specifically note if the behaviour was dangerous and if the child's will to die was strong. Note the presence of a detailed plan, the taking of precautions to avoid discovery and the carrying out of a final act like making a will or writing a note.

If you are reassessing a youngster who has been hospitalized with a view to discharging the case, or if you are assessing a case where suicide is suspected but no self-injurious behaviour has occurred, ask these questions.

- *Have you thought of harming yourself?*
- *How strong is the urge to harm yourself?*
- *Have you a plan to harm yourself?*
- *What preparations have you made to harm yourself?*
- *Suppose, you harmed yourself and died, what do you hope your family/your mum/your dad/your brother/your sister would think/do/feel?*
- *Suppose, you harmed yourself but didn't die, what do you hope your family/your mum/your dad/your brother/your sister would think/do/feel?*
- *Do you want to escape from something or some situation?*
- *Do you want to punish somebody by harming yourself?*

Note if the plan includes specific details of a dangerous method, precautions against discovery and a final act such as writing a suicide note or a will. The Beck Scale for Suicide Ideation is a useful adjunct to a clinical interview (Beck, 1991).

3. Establish the circumstances surrounding the episode

In cases where an attempt has been made, build up a picture of the immediate circumstances surrounding the episode; what happened before, during and after the episode? Clarify if this is a escalation of an entrenched pattern of interaction around previous suicidal ideas or intentions.

In cases where no self-injury has occurred but where suicidal ideation is present, ask the youngster to describe the sequence of events that lead up to and follow on from episodes of suicidal ideation.

4. Explore risk factors in the social network

Identify the youngsters perception of the network and their perception of the roles of significant people in the recent episode and previous episodes. Include family, friends and involved professionals in this assessment. The procedures for constructing and elaborating a genogram and lifeline described earlier may be useful here.

Use the genogram and lifeline to explore the following risk factors: social isolation, crowding, recent stressful life events or losses and criticism or abuse of the child by members of the network. Social isolation due to social mobility rather than family death or the family growing up and moving away is more common among parasuicide cases than are completed suicides. Crowding and long term unemployment are also more common among parasuicidal cases. Recent stressful life events and losses of particular relevance to children and adolescents include loss of a family member or friend through death, hospitalisation, emigration, unwanted pregnancy; loss of health; loss of status; exam failure and expected exam failure. In distinguishing between suicide and parasuicide, it is worth noting that separation through family disruption, court appearance, personal illness and illness in the family are more commonly associated with parasuicide. In distinguishing between suicide and parasuicide, rejection following angry quarrels between youngsters and their girlfriends or boyfriends is more common among parasuicides. (Also on the theme of rejection, parents with children in care, due to chaotic family management, are over-represented among adult parasuicidal cases.)

5. Identify psychological, medical and demographic predisposing factors

Once a clear understanding of the suicidal ideation, intent and behaviour have been clarified and placed within the context of a pattern of social interaction, move on to clarify the presence of psychological, medical and demographic characteristics that may predispose the youngster to self-harm. What follows is a brief discussion of each of some of the more important predisposing psychological, medical and demographic risk factors around which clinicians should base their inquires in Positive Practice.

The first and most important to consider is a history of previous self-harm. Such a history is associated with both suicide and parasuicide. In the year following deliberate self harm, the risk of suicide is 1 to 2%. This is 100 times higher than in the normal population. When an individualistic psychiatric diagnosis based on a system like DSM IV (APA, 1994) or ICD 10 (WHO, 1992) is made, it has been found that major depression is uniquely associated with suicide and dysthymia or minor depression with parasuicide. Major depression within the DSM classification system is characterized by at least five of the following symptoms: low mood, loss of interest in all activities, significantly reduced or increased appetite, insomnia or hypersomnia, psychomotor retardation or agitation, loss of energy, feelings of worthlessness, diminished concentration, and recurrent thoughts of death. Minor depression is characterized by low mood and at least two of the symptoms listed. Major depression tends to be episodic, whereas minor depression tends to be chronic. However, it is important to emphasize that while these disorders are constructed by a community of mental health practitioners and scientists in individualistic terms, both phenomena may also be constructed as segments of broader interactional patterns (Tomm, 1991).

Chronic rather than experimental alcohol and drug use are both risk factors for both suicide and parasuicide so these are important areas deserving inquiry in cases of self harm. Extreme antisocial behaviour in older teenagers is probably a risk factor for parasuicide. This is based on the finding that, in adults, antisocial personality disorder (as defined in the DSM or ICD diagnostic systems) is present in one-third to one-half of parasuicide cases. Adults with antisocial personality disorders usually have a history of conduct disorders as children and delinquent or criminal features present in adolescence or early adulthood. They typically have come from chaotic families, have poor internalised standards of behaviour, and show poor impulse control.

Chronic painful illness is associated with completed suicide, and the incidence of suicide is four times the average among people with epilepsy.

Suicide is more common among men than women whereas parasuicide is more common among women. In many countries including Ireland, the incidence of suicide among young males (18 to 25) has increased dramatically over the past decade. Parasuicide is associated with the fifteen to twenty-five year age group.

The risk of suicide is highest in extreme socio-economic groups. That is, among those from families where the parents are unskilled workers or unemployed on the one hand, or are higher professionals or senior managers on the other. Parasuicide occurs most commonly in lower socio-economic groups.

The risks of suicide and parasuicide are associated with marital status. Of particular importance in assessing adolescents is the finding that parasuicide is more common among teenage wives. Finally, the incidence of suicide varies with the season and is most common in early summer (April, May and June in this hemisphere).

6. Identify protective factors

A crucial part of the individual consultation is to explore factors that the child perceives may contribute to a solution which is an alternative to suicide. These include, untapped positive relationships with significant network members; a personal openness to checking out opportunities to talk through conflictual issues with parents, teachers, foster parents friends or other significant network members; and an openness to exploring factors related to the wish to live and the wish to die. Here are some useful questions to ask in exploring protective factors.

- *At the moment it seems to you as if there is no way out. I wonder when you look at the genogram you have drawn, if there is anyone on it who you suspect might be able to help you now?*
- *One of the main things that seems to be trapping you is the belief that your father/mother/teacher/ friend will do X to you if you do Y. Just say there was an opportunity to check that out. Would you be willing to ask them to spell out what they would do and what they think about it?*
- *It sounds like one part of you wants to end your life now. But you would not still be living, if there was not another part of you that wants to continue living. I'm curious about what sort of things seem to be making that part of you want to keep living?*

7. Integrate the child's story, check its accuracy and agree a plan for discussing this account with members of the network

Sandra was a seventeen year old girl who developed post-traumatic stress disorder following an incident where she was attacked and robbed. Her parents and herself participated in a series of consultations and within this context developed a way to cope with the nightmares, intrusive thoughts and emotions and sense of threat that Sandra experienced. Eventually the symptoms disappeared. Six months after the family ended therapy, the parents phoned seeking an urgent appointment for Sandra who had threatened to take an overdose. As part of the consultation process to the family, I saw Sandra on her own and conducted an individual suicide risk assessment along the lines set out in this chapter. This interview was concluded with the following integration and plan for feedback.

"Let me just pull this whole thing together now to see if I've understood you right, OK. You say, on Thursday you felt so down that you thought it would be easier to take a lot of pills and kill yourself than to go on living. You say that you thought this because you had started to get nightmares a week ago.... about person who attacked and robbed you again and you had bad feelings during the day. The nightmares and the bad feelings made you think each day...'I can't take it....I've got to escape...' After a week of nightmares, followed by bad feelings, followed by thoughts of escape... in the end you thought the way out was to take an overdose. This cycle started up following three big changes in your life that have all just come together. The first was your Nan's death last month. The second was going back to school into your final year where the exam pressure is on. The third was you feeling like you were trapped in your relationship with Terry (your boyfriend) and you can't get out but you know you have to. When I draw this sort of explanation out this is what it looks like (Figure 14.7). Have I understood you right? This minute, you say the part of you that wants to live is stronger than the part of you that wants to die. Have I got that right? Now, it seems to me that your parents will be able to back you up best if they understand that and know about this map here (Figure 14.7). Is it OK with you if I go over this explanation with them? The other thing is this... If you could have some way of talking about the bad feelings, the nightmares and the sense of being unsafe during the day at school....then it would make it easier for you and you say that you would feel less like using an overdose as a way to escape. You want to see if Miss Chadwick would let you visit her if need be."

In this case Sharon agreed to sharing this construction of the problem and a possible solution with her parents. The parents threw light on their role in the cycle of interaction around the problem. For example, they both said that the grandmother's death had made them less available to Sharon and less sensitive to the fact that the relapse was a serious concern for her. These factors were built into the three column formulation. A plan was developed which included Sharon being able to visit the teacher with whom she had a special relationship (Miss Chadwick) during school hours, or being able to phone home. Weekly follow-up consultations were offered, and these were used to help Sharon cope with her nightmares and for the therapist to support her parents.

In cases where youngsters request that some aspect of the summary of their account of the circumstances surrounding the suicidal ideation, intention or behaviour be kept confidential, the confidentiality should only be disregarded if keeping it will place the youngster at risk, and preclude the development of a workable solution for the youngster and the family. In cases where children have been abused, neglected or are involved in drug abuse, prostitution or other dangerous activity, decision making about confidentiality is complex. The risk reducing benefits of breaking confidentiality need to be balanced against the negative impact of this on the youngster's perception of the therapist as a trustworthy adult, and the dangers of maintaining confidentiality and leaving the child in a potentially risky situation need to be balanced against the benefits of maintaining a trusting therapeutic alliance. Sharing these dilemmas with a team or supervisor is an important part of Positive Practice. The management of ethical dilemmas is discussed in Chapter 17.

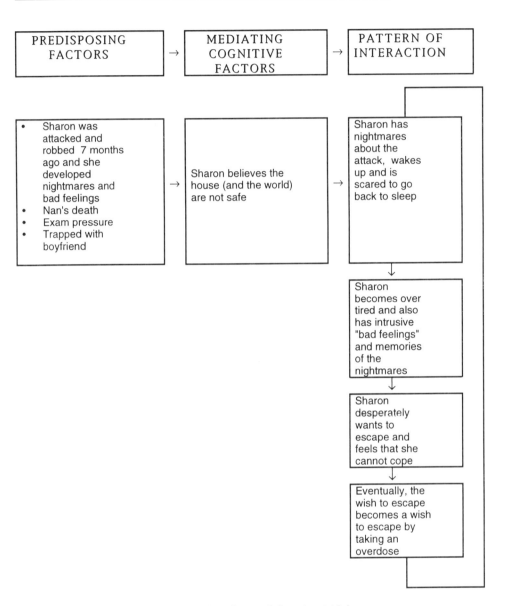

Figure 14.7.   Preliminary three column formulation of Sharon's suicidal thoughts based on an individual interview

SUMMARY AND COMMENTS

The virtual exclusion of children from family therapy is unfortunately a common practice. In a major US survey Korner and Brown (1990) found that 40% of therapists excluded children from therapy sessions and 31% only included them in a token way. This is a serious problem. In Positive Practice, particular care is taken to provide youngsters with space to be heard in the family consultation process. Individual consultations are one avenue through which this is achieved.

Individual consultations may fruitfully be used within Positive Practice to assess children's views and abilities, to help children develop skills or evolve new belief systems and to offer the child a forum in which to be heard at times of crisis. Such crises include situations where abuse is suspected or where there is a risk of self-harm or violence to others.

In Positive Practice, individual consultations must be planned within a systemic context. There should be a clear set of objectives for individual consultations. The way of working within the consultation should clearly address the objectives of the consultations. There should be agreement on the limits of confidentiality and the degree to which information from the individual consultations may be shared and the way in which this is fed back into family meetings. The roles of child advocate or key worker and consultant to the family and wider system must be clearly differentiated and negotiated within the treatment system. There must be clear agreements on the way in which information from the individual consultation is fed back into larger family or network meetings.

Where children present with threats of self-harm or self-injurious behaviour the first step in an individual consultation is to clarify the youngster's expectations and the limits of confidentiality. This should be followed with an exploration of the details of the child's suicidal ideation, suicidal intention and self-injurious behaviour. Then the circumstances surrounding the episode require clarification and risk factors in the social network may be explored. From there, move on to identify the psychological, medical and demographic predisposing factors and also identify protective factors. Finally, integrate the child's story, check its accuracy and agree a plan for discussing this account with members of the network.

Exercise 14.1

Work in pairs.

One person take the role of therapist and the other take the role of a child in a family on their current case load.

The person taking the role of the child must first brief the therapist on the circumstances surrounding the referral.

During the role-play, the therapist must conduct a child-centred assessment following the guidelines set out in this chapter and summarized in Figure 14.1.

Derole after the exercise.

Take 20 minutes to discuss
1.   The experience of the person who took the role of the child
2.   The areas in which the therapist felt competent and the areas in which the therapist felt
        challenged when conducting the child centred assessment.

Exercise 14.2.

Work in pairs.

One person take the role of therapist and the other take the role of Karen White (whom we first met in Exercise 13.2.).

Karen requests an individual appointment when the family arrive at the clinic the day after the crisis meeting with John (mentioned in Exercise 13.2). During this interview she has had thoughts about slashing her wrists.

The person role-playing the therapist must conduct a full self-harm assessment following the guidelines set out in this chapter.

Derole after the exercise.

Take 20 minutes to discuss
1.   The experience of Karen during the interview
2.   The areas in which the therapist felt competent and the areas in which the therapist felt
        challenged when managing the self-harm assessment.

15

Network Meetings

In the Barrow Case, the individual consultation with Caroline was followed by a network meeting. In this chapter, the process and outcome of this meeting will be reviewed and some general guidelines for convening network meetings will be given.

You will remember that the network meeting was held two days after the crisis phonecall. The following people attended: Dick, Sheila and Caroline Barrow; the GP, Dr Wilson; the school nurse, Sarah Boyd; the EWO Phil Hutchinson and the year-head Ms Hackett. The Paediatrician Dr Tom Walker was invited but was unavailable. Because of his peripheral involvement in the case, his absence was not sufficient to postpone the meeting. However, he did say to me in a telephone conversation prior to the network meeting that he was firmly of the view that Caroline's abdominal pains were not symptomatic of an organic gastrointestinal disorder. He also said that if the outcome of the meeting was that a further examination of Caroline were required he would be happy to oblige. The Clinical Medical Officer (school doctor), Dr Reid, was also unavailable. However, he was represented by the school nurse, Sarah Boyd, and both Sarah and Dr Reid usually took the same position on case management decisions, so Dr Reid's absence was not a deterrent to proceeding with the meeting. David Trellis, the Educational Psychologist who referred the case was no longer involved because he had changed jobs and his post had not been filled since his transfer.

Had the GP or a representative of the school been unavailable, the network meeting would have encountered difficulties in developing a plan to manage Caroline's difficulties which were construed by the professional network as having both medical and educational dimensions.

The network meeting began with introductions. The GP, Dr Wilson, was pleased to meet the school nurse, Sarah Boyd and the year head Ms Hackett. Dick and Sheila were being introduced to the school nurse for the first time. So, for some members of the network, the introductions process was a way of connecting with members of the network that they had not previously met. For Caroline, it was a somewhat threatening experience because it was the first time so many of the adults who were concerned with her difficulties had come together in one place to talk about her. Some weeks after the meeting in the final session, she said that she felt desperately embarrassed by the whole affair and she wished everyone would just leave her alone.

Following introductions, I summarized the case as follows and set the agenda for the meeting. "Caroline was referred here by Dr Tom Walker, the Paediatrician and David Trellis, the Educational Psychologist ....who eh.. Most of us know ...in the middle of February, about eight months ago. There were two sides to the problem. The first is that Caroline regularly experiences......about three times a week at least now...... strong stomach pains. The second is that these are sometimes so bad that she is unable to attend school. All of us here have seen one or other or both sides of the problem.. at one time or another. These pains prevent Caroline from doing things that she wants to do.......But medical tests done by the Paediatrician, Dr Tom Walker....... and yourself, Dr Wilson, show that the pains are not due to a physical illness, an infection, a tumour, or some internal injury or other......I suppose they hold this ... in common with headaches.....no physical illness but a genuine experience of pain. It seems that the pains are worst in the morning and are exacerbated by eh...by discussing them at that time. It also seems that they become less intense when Caroline is engrossed in things like schoolwork, housework or conversations with people who she sees as on her side and who do not focus on the pain issue. However....these conclusions are only tentative.

Recently, I guess we have all been trying to coordinate our efforts to help Caroline but .....well....we have come to a full stop. On Monday....Caroline found herself.... almost beaten by the pains.... unable to go to school at all. She has been at home since. Today's meeting is a chance for us all to look for a way out of this situation so that the pain can be managed and Caroline can return to school. That's the agenda for today. We have about an hour. So lets begin. Let's run it so that each of us presents our view and then, in about forty minutes, we take a breather. Then reconvene when we have had a chance to collect our thoughts and formulate a fairly focused plan for the next step to take."

I then asked Sheila what her main concern was now. She said that she still believed that some medical problem had been missed and she elaborated this in some detail. I put this to Dr Wilson who said that there was no evidence to support this although he agreed that the pain was present and could be anxiety related or a reflection of an underlying depression. Nurse Boyd agreed with this and expanded on other school based signs that Caroline may be depressed or anxious about some unknown events. I acknowledged to Sheila that it was difficult to be in a situation where your heart told you that Caroline possibly had cancer but where the medical evidence did not appear to support this. I pointed out that the possibility of a second opinion being offered by Dr Walker the Paediatrician remained open as a way of addressing Sheila's dilemma.

I then asked Dick about his chief concerns. He said that he believed originally that Caroline was disobedient and malingering but now, following the crisis on Monday, he thought that she might be disturbed and in need of medication and hospitalisation. I asked him to expand on this, which he did, and he concluded by saying that he really wanted to know what a full assessment of Caroline as an individual would reveal. I then explained to the meeting that I had responded to this request by conducting a full assessment of Caroline before the network meeting and that, in my role as someone who was advocating for Caroline on an individual basis, I would present my findings to the meeting. I said that the psychological evaluation I had conducted before the network meeting showed that Caroline was upset but not psychologically disturbed. I acknowledged that she must have looked like she was not herself on Monday when she attacked him after he insisted that she go to school. I confirmed that there was no evidence of psychosis or suicidal intent. I mentioned that a second opinion could be sought from another psychologist or psychiatrist if Caroline showed further clear signs of bizarre behaviour. Dick was reluctant for more professionals to become involved.

The school teacher, Ms Hackett, then confirmed that she saw Caroline's behaviour as a reflection of her being worried about something, rather than being disturbed or mentally ill. She said that she was prepared to make herself available to Caroline as a sounding-board if that would be helpful.

I then asked Caroline if she could tell the meeting how she would like to progress. She said she just wanted to be left alone. She said that she did not want to see any more doctors. I asked if she wanted to use the meeting to negotiate an agreement with her parents, her teacher, Dr Wilson and Nurse Boyd where she could plan her own return to school and her pain management programme. She agreed to this.

I asked how she would like to arrange things and, with only a little facilitation, Caroline outlined the following plan. She said that she would like to go to school every day. If she felt sick or had stomachaches she did not want anyone to ask her about it. Then, once in school, she wanted permission to leave class if the pains were so bad that could not concentrate. But she did not want anyone hassling her about it. She wanted to be able to talk to Ms Hackett from time to time, but not on an appointment basis.

Everyone involved agreed to the plan and the Barrows were offered a follow-up appointment for the following Thursday. No break was taken during the meeting to collect thoughts and come up with a plan since none appeared to be necessary.

GUIDELINES FOR CONVENING NETWORK MEETINGS

Network meetings may be convened for a variety of reasons. They are most usefully convened when a therapeutic system is in a state of transition or extreme stuckness. In the Barrow case, the transition was marked by the emergence of the therapeutic crisis. When a worker accepts a new referral, or where new management in an agency requires each case to be reviewed, often network meetings are highly appropriate. Network meetings may also be called when cases become particularly stuck (Carpenter and Treacher, 1989).

1. Set clear goals

The context within which the network meeting is called, be it transition or stuckness, will have implications for the goals of the meeting. In cases where the clinician is stuck or new to the case, the network meeting may be convened with the goal of identifying the main customer and clarifying the consultation contract; identifying the most useful system to work with for the process of formulation construction; constructing a formulation; or meeting others who may have resources that would be useful in implementing a solution that follows from a formulation. Methods for mapping out the roles network members play in the problem-system so as to avoid engagement mistakes have already been described in Chapter 2. The issue of who to invite to network meetings will be discussed in the next section.

In crises, where a clear formulation is guiding the consultation process, goals are set in the light of the formulation. In the Barrow case, the central goal of the meeting was to develop a plan to help Caroline manage pain and to attend school and to arrange this with a shared interactional construction of the problem. The setting of the goals for the meeting was informed by the overall three column formulation set out in Figure 7.1. These primary goals were set within the context of a crisis in which Mr Barrow had pushed for an individualistic reformulation of Caroline's difficulties. In some instances it may be useful to begin by recapping the overall three column formulation that has been guiding the consultation process.

Where therapists fail to convene network meetings at critical points in the consultation process, or where they call meetings without a clear plan and procedure for managing the meeting, usually the process of problem resolution is compromised. Had the meeting not been called, there was a strong probability that someone in the Barrow family would draw one or more network members into the cycle of interaction around the problem to confirm an individualistic problem formulation in the manner outlined in Figure 13.3.

Clear goals are a critical feature of network meetings. Meetings without clear goals are often destructive, particularly when professionals' sense of uncertainty about the meeting and the case lead them to experience anxiety and this becomes channelled into confrontative or competitive interactions with other network members. This is particularly apt to happen in multiproblem cases where risks of abuse or self-harm are potentially present. Often these dangerous goalless meetings lead professionals into polarized positions characterized by the countertransference reactions discussed in Chapter 11. Inevitably such polarized professional networks develop an organizational structure which mirrors that of the family around which the professionals are organized (McCarthy and Byrne, 1988). Of course, having a framework within which to conceptualize the development of such dysfunctional patterns of organization is helpful to orient a therapist towards clear network meeting goals. A number of useful frameworks for mapping out alliances and countertransference reactions which lead to polarization will be presented later in the chapter.

2. Decide who to invite

In Chapter 2, principles to guide decisions about who to invite to intake interviews were outlined. Similar principles are useful in deciding who to invite to a network meeting. The decision should be based upon an analysis of the roles played by the members of the network. These roles include the referring agent, the customer, the problem person, those legally responsible for the problem person, the primary caretakers, system members who promote stuckness and system members who promote change. The customer must be present at the network meeting and the legal guardian of the referred child must have given consent for the meeting to go ahead. Ideally, the youngster identified as the problem person and the primary caretakers should also be present. Where an infant is the main reason for referral, it may be more productive to hold the meeting without the problem person. Where agents of social control, such as statutory social workers or probation officers are involved or potentially involved, they should also be present. Referring agents should also be included .

There is little point progressing with the meeting unless the customer and the legal guardian of the child and the involved agent of social control are present since no meaningful decisions can then be made. Where any of these key network members are absent the meeting should be brief and its focus should be on identifying a way of convening a network meeting with all key members present.

3. Open with introductions

Often network meetings are the first time network members have met. Because of this, introductions are vital. Encourage members to identify themselves and their role in the case and to state who they know and who they do not know. Here is an example of how to open a network meeting.

- *Hello. Thank you all for coming here today. Let's start with introductions since some of us are meeting for the first time. I'm Alan Carr. I'm the Clinical Psychologist here ......eh ...at this unit. I've known Sheila and Dick and .....Caroline for about two months now. They originally came to me at Tom Walker's request. ....He's the paediatrician in the district hospital as most of you know. David Trellis, the educational psychologist also wrote at the same time asking me to offer Caroline an appointment. I've spoken to all of you on the phone this week. But its my first time meeting you Ms Hackett. Its good to meet you in person. ....Would you eh.. like to introduce yourself now ? Tell us what your involvement is and which of us you know?*

Introductions are a forum within which certain important distinctions may be made. At the close of the introductions section of the meeting it should be clear to all participants who the family members are, who the professionals are, and who other involved people are, such as foster parents or befrienders. It should also be clear to everyone which professionals have statutory responsibility for the case and which professionals do not. Introductions also throw light on the degree of involvement of each person with the problem.

A second function of the introduction process is to provide a forum where network members who do not know each other can take the first step towards forming a working alliance.

4. Set the agenda and the rules for participation

In the Barrow case, the goal of the meeting was stated as finding a way to help Caroline handle the pain and the school attendance problem. Confusion can be greatly reduced in network meetings by stating the overall goal or objectives clearly at the outset. A number of goals are commonly addressed in network meetings. Where clinicians are new to a case, often the goal of a network meeting is to clarify who the main customer is and what exactly her or she wishes to achieve through the process of consultation (Dimmock and Dungworth, 1985). If this has been clarified but the case is either stuck or in crisis, the goal of the network meeting may be to construct or elaborate a formulation, or to evolve a plan.

Each person is then given an opportunity by the convenor to outline their involvement in some detail, to state their concerns and to give their opinion in relation to the stated goal of the meeting. This process of providing space for each person to tell the story of the case from their position offers multiple perspectives on the problem and various approaches to its resolution, the patterns of alliances or coalitions within the overall network, the belief systems from which network members are operating and countertransference reactions that involved professionals may be experiencing. These issues will be discussed in more detail below.

The convenor also sets the time frame and the time structure. The structure that I intended to use for the Barrow case is a useful framework. That is, to work for about forty to sixty minutes and then to break for about fifteen minutes so that everyone, especially the convenor, can collect their thoughts before presenting a tentative integration of the material discussed and options for action that may serve as the basis for a plan.

5. Make sure everyone gets a fair hearing

No matter how clearly the structure is set, two problems typically emerge in meetings. Some people say too much and others say little or nothing. A crucial part of the convenor's role is to help over-talkative people to condense what they have to say into a succinct verbal nugget and to help the reticent members of the network to elaborate their positions. Here is an example of how to deal with someone who has a lot to say.

- *You've said X and Y. This will be useful to all of us in looking for a way through these difficulties. You have a lot more to tell us about this problem. But time is tight. So I'm wondering if you could take a couple of minutes to reflect on the top three things that we would need to know as a group in order to use your knowledge to help us solve the central problem we are focusing on today. That is, the problem of XYZ.*

Here is an example of how to help someone increase their contribution to a meeting.

- *I guess that you may know more about this than many of us, so can you give us some examples to show us why you believe XYZ?*

Where a youngster's position is being represented to the group by an advocate it is important that this be flagged. For example, with the Barrows I said the following.

- *Today I'm wearing two hats. One of my jobs is to chair this meeting in a neutral sort of way and to take no one's side. However, I also took on the job of doing a psychological assessment with Caroline to clarify her position in some detail and she asked me to act as her advocate and present the outcome of this individual session to the meeting.*

6. Use summarizing to help members maintain focus

People's concentration may wax and wane throughout a meeting. Anxiety and boredom both interfere with our capacity to concentrate on all that is said in network meetings. To help everyone maintain focus, it is the convenor's role to summarize periodically what has been said. A useful technique is to keep some brief notes and periodically condense these into point form or diagrammatic form on a flipchart or whiteboard.

7. Maintain neutrality

In order to help all group members represent their positions clearly, the convenor must retain a neutral position where he or she does not appear to side with any one person or faction. Neutrality involves taking sides with no one against anyone else; operating from a position of respectful curiosity about each person's perspective on the problem; challenging everyone to elaborate the patterns of behaviour that they see related to the problem and its resolution and the beliefs that they hold about these, and, most importantly challenging everyone to move from an individualistic framing of the problem to an interactional framing (Selvini-Palazzoli et al, 1980a; Cecchin, 1987).

8. Integrate the results of the meeting and devise a plan

When everyone in the network meeting has been given an opportunity to address the problem, the convenor may find it valuable to take time out for a few minutes to integrate the emerging constructions of the problem and its resolution into a formulation from which a clear action plan may be derived. Some clinicians may wish to share this responsibility with the entire network meeting. The advantages and disadvantages of formulating complex material privately or openly has already been discussed in Chapter 7 with reference to active interactional cotherapy (Hoffman and Gafni, 1984) and reflecting teams (Andersen, 1989). My own preference is to take time to formulate, especially if the network meeting occurs during a crisis and members of the network are polarizing into extreme emotional positions. Time out provides space to think clearly. The simpler the formulation and the plan the better. However, it is important that the formulation retain an interactional rather than an individualistic construction of the problem. I have found that a full three column formulation is commonly too complex to present in full network meetings, so often a condensed version of it is presented along with some options for action. Often it will become obvious with the network meeting that one or more professionals are about to be or have been sucked into the pattern of interaction around the presenting problem in a way that maintains rather than dissolves this cycle. In such instances, the interactional formulation of the problem must include this.

9. Discuss the formulation and optional plans and agree on a course of action

After time-out, present the formulation and optional action plans. These must be presented tentatively with room for members of the network to suggest minor modifications. Once they have been accepted, ask all members if they would like to formulate a short term plan so that everybody will be clear on their role and responsibilities within the network. This is a form of contracting that facilitates the closing of the meeting. Once there is support for the idea of developing a plan, check which optional plan each member would favour. Finally, explore ways in which responsibilities may be allocated. In the Barrow case this process was short circuited, with Caroline pushing for her preferred solution quite early in the proceedings before a reformulation of the problem and related action plans were formally presented to the meeting. This is not uncommon and often bodes well for the outcome of the case.

In child protection cases a clear distinction may usefully be made between the monitoring and support functions. One solution to working with families where a statutory child protection order is in place is for the statutory social worker alone, to retain the function of monitoring the family's status with respect to clearly stated safety criteria. Another professional or group of professionals may explicitly take on the role of empowering the family to meet these criteria (Crowther et al, 1990).

It may be helpful to all network members, particularly where the plan is complex, to agree to send all members of the network a succinct summary of the key points of the action plan. Such letters may include a list of all involved parties, the central customer in the network who required your involvement, the central problem with which the customer wants help, the question addressed in the network meeting, the allocation of tasks that was agreed at the meeting and a review date if one was settled upon. A letter sent to those involved in the Barrow case is contained in Figure 15.1. A summary of guidelines for convening network meetings is set out in Figure 15.2.

PARTICIPATING IN NETWORK MEETINGS

To participate productively in a network meeting, prepare well before you arrive and make a list of some or all of the following points, stating each one as concisely as possible.

1. Your own involvement in the case and how you see yourself connected into the network of professionals working with the case
2. Your agency's previous involvement in the case
3. The terms of reference of your agency's and your own involvement in the case
4. Your view of the main concerns at present
5. Your hypothesis about the current difficulties
6. Your view of possible solutions to the problems
7. The possible contribution that yourself and your agency may make and the limits of your potential future involvement.

Use the slack period while waiting for late-comers to turn up to the meeting to build relationships with those members of the network with whom you are *least* familiar. This informal contact helps to build the sort of working alliances that help network members work together flexibly and reduces the probability of polarisation. (Polarization and other difficulties are discussed in more detail below.)

If the person who is convening the meeting omits formal introductions from the proceedings, when you are asked to make your contribution, begin by introducing yourself to network members with whom you are unfamiliar and offer them a chance to introduce themselves to you. This increases the informality of the meeting and relaxes an often tense atmosphere.

Use your first speaking turn to make points about your own involvement in the case and that of your agency. Sometimes it is useful to wait until everyone at the meeting has presented information on their involvement before offering your hypothesis and ideas about solutions.

When you present the story of your own and your agency's involvement conclude with a clear summary of the key points.

When the convenor moves on to discuss ways of formulating the problem and possible solutions, indicate clearly that your have something to say about the matter. This is particularly important if you are a junior professional or a trainee. When you are invited to contribute, make your points succinctly. Present your own hypotheses tentatively. Acknowledge the limits of your own and your agency's potential future involvement in the case.

Child and Family Clinic
Market Town
Norfolk

Re: The Barrows

A network meeting took place on 5.4.90.

The following people attended: Caroline, Dick and Sheila Barrow; Dr Wilson (GP); Nurse Boyd; Phil Hutchinson (EWO) and Ms Hackett (school nurse at Lowlands High School).
The following sent their apologies: Dr Tom Walker (Paediatrician) and Dr Reed (CMO)

The meeting was called in response to Dick and Sheila's concern over Caroline's abdominal pains and school attendance difficulties. These problems have been ongoing for over a year despite Trojan efforts on the part of all members of the family and network to find a workable solution.

According to both Dr Walker and Dr Wilson, the pains are not due to organic factors. Our psychological assessment of the problem suggests that these severe pains, much like tension headaches, seem to be maintained by the patterns of interaction that Caroline has with important people in her life.

It was agreed at the meeting that Caroline take control of her own pain management and return to school programme, and that she be supported by all of us in this.

When at school, Ms Hackett agreed to make herself available to Caroline as a sounding board as the need arises.

No review network meeting was planned. However, follow up appointments at our unit were scheduled for Caroline and her parents and if the need arises further network meetings will be called.

Thank you all for your help and cooperation.

Yours sincerely

Alan Carr
Clinical Psychologist

Figure 15.1. Letter sent to network members following a network meeting

CONVENING NETWORK MEETINGS

1. Set the goal
2. Decide who to invite
3. Open with introductions
4. Set the agenda and the rules for participation
5. Make sure everyone gets a fair hearing
6. Summarize periodically
7. Retain neutrality
8. Formulate and plan options
9. Agree a course of action

Figure 15.2. Guidelines for network meetings

If observations or hypotheses about the case offered by other members are at variance with your observations or hypotheses, present your viewpoint to the convenor rather than to the person with whom you disagree. Emphasize the specific events that have led you to form a different viewpoint. No matter how strongly you feel about your own position and how much negative emotion you feel about the person with whom you disagree, focus on clarifying the issue not on attacking the colleague or client with whom you disagree.

Do not leave a network meeting without clearly establishing what is the next step yourself and your agency have agreed to take with respect to the case.

Write a note into the casefile following the meeting. Specify who attended, what overall formulation was agreed and what role each professional, including yourself, agreed to take in future.

If a network meeting leaves you with strong ambivalent feelings, make a point of discussing the meeting informally with a trusted colleague or in a supervision meeting with your clinical supervisor.

The approach to participating in network meetings outlined here, and summarized in Figure 15.3, may also be useful in contributing to wardrounds, case conferences or multidisciplinary team meetings.

CONTRIBUTING TO NETWORK MEETINGS

1.	Prepare points on your involvement, your hypotheses and plans
2.	Build working alliances during slack time
3.	Always introduce yourself before making your first contribution
4.	Outline your involvement first and hypotheses and plans second
5.	Make your points briefly
6.	Summarize your points at the end of each major contribution
7.	When you disagree, focus on clarifying the issue not on attacking the person
8.	Write down who attended, the formulation and the plan in the casefile
9.	Discuss unresolved ambivalent feelings in supervision

Figure 15.3.   Guidelines for contributing to network meetings

PROBLEMS IN NETWORK MEETINGS

A frequent problem with network meetings is the development of cooperation difficulties. Whether you are convening or contributing to a network meeting, it is vital to have a way of understanding cooperation difficulties. Such problems may be analysed in terms of behavioural sequences, polarized beliefs that network members hold, polarized countertransference reactions and patterns of alliances. Let us examine each of these in turn.

Mapping Out Behavioural Sequences

A common difficulty that occurs in network meetings is where the professional network on the one hand and the family on the other develop either a rigid symmetrical relationship or a rigid complimentary relationship. (These two types of relationships were previously mentioned in Chapter 3 when we explored ways of mapping out patterns of interaction around a presenting problem.) Typical examples of symmetrical and complimentary relationships are set out in Figure 15.4. In the example of the symmetrical relationship the more professionals offer help, the more the family members provide reasons why this help will be of no value. In transactional analysis this pattern of interaction is called the *Yes but...game* (Dusay and Dusay, 1989). The clients ask for help, but when it is offered in a variety of forms, the clients point out reasons why they cannot cooperate with the helping process by saying "Yes but...." Within network meetings it is important to describe and question the symmetrical escalation process and the beliefs that underpin it.

- *It appears that there is a difficulty in matching the help that is on offer to the needs of Mary, Tom and Barbara. So rather than go on with trying to put together a plan, lets back-pedal a bit and explore what help would look like to Barbara, Mary and Tom if they got it, and what good help means....*
- *Barbara, can you guess what good help would look like to Tom?*
- *What belief do you think Tom has that makes him think X is helpful/unhelpful?*

This circular questioning process may be continued until it is clear what beliefs underpin the symmetrical escalation. When these are clear, the best way to offer help and more importantly, the way not to offer help will become apparent.

In network meetings, complimentary relationships are most noticeable where offers of help by involved professionals are eagerly accepted and followed by requests for even more help. Where complimentary relationships develop between a family and a professional network in the field, the more help the professionals offer the more problems the family present. This type of relationship is diagrammed in Figure 15.4. The complimentary pattern may be acknowledged in a network meeting, and circular

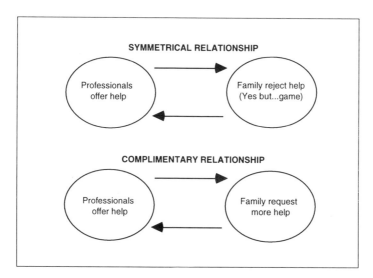

Figure 15.4.   Simple symmetrical and complimentary relationships between families and members of the professional network

questioning may focus on the limits of the resources and the limits of the family's needs and their beliefs about the helping process.

- *There seems to be a problem here with deciding about how much help to give and what sort of help this should be. You (to clients) need sufficient advice to help you deal with XYZ and I've been listening to valiant attempts by those involved to put together a package to meet this need. But every time it looks like the package is in place, the idea that it is not enough recurs and so it has to be revamped. Let's take a bit of time to look at that.*
- *Tom, ideally, how do you think things at your house would look, if the group here were able to give yourself and the two boys (two mentally handicapped children aged twelve and fourteen years) all the help you need?*
- *How would you know if you had received too much help?*
- *How do you see the responsibilities for the care of your boys being divided up between yourself and the district handicap team?*
- *What beliefs about education and health care inform your view?*

Mapping Out Ideas

In any network meeting an ecology of ideas or beliefs emerges from members' contributions. With the Barrows, it was clear that the idea that Caroline's symptoms could be construed as either of *organic* or *non-organic* aetiology was central to the networks discourse about the problem. Sheila saw the problem as being of organic aetiology while Dr Wilson and Nurse Boyd saw the aetiology as non-organic. A second construct that was used by the network in making sense of Caroline's difficulties was that of *badness* versus *madness*. Dick originally saw the problem as primarily one of disobedience, malingering and Caroline being essentially *bad*. However, following the crisis, he reconstrued her as mentally ill or *mad*.

Identifying and mapping out these bipolar constructs is a very useful aid to managing conflicting views which emerge in a network meeting. Imelda Colgan (1991) and her colleagues from the fifth Province team show how such pairs of significant bipolar constructs may be used to form diamond- shaped maps like that presented in Figure 15.5. Such maps may be used as a basis for questioning network members in a way that moves the network towards a position where less polarization occurs. Two approaches to questions developed by the fifth Province team deserve particular mention. These are questioning at the extremes and juxtapositioning. In questioning at the extremes, the network member is asked to imagine what would happen if one of the extreme positions on the diamond were to form the basis for future actions. Here are some examples.

- *Let's say we agreed today that her behaviour was fundamentally an act of defiance and that she required some form of punishment. Can you say what sort of things we should all do and say if she continued to appear defiant over the next three years?*
- *You are thinking that this may reflect some underlying mental illness. If that were so how would you see things panning out over the next year or so, if you did what was necessary to care for her. That is, if you treated her as if he was mentally ill?*
- *If this were depression here. If your partner were wracked with grief for reasons that we cannot fully understand now. How would she manage over the next year and how would you and the rest of the family deal with her as a person debilitated by grief?*

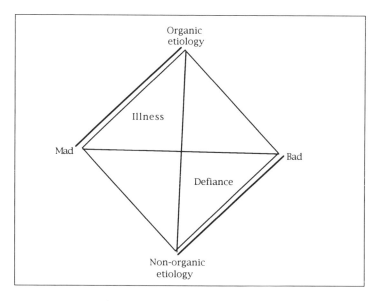

Figure 15.5.   Diamond map of constructs used by the network to construe Caroline's symptoms

Questioning at the extremes is obviously a technique which allows network members to explore what would happen if a process of continual *amplification* occurred with respect to their construction of the problem. With juxtapositioning, the network member is asked to consider the belief systems that underpin opposing positions on the diamond or the behaviours and emotions associated with them.

- *Your sister's view seems to be X. Your partner's view differs from that. She is saying Y. What do you see as the main differences between the beliefs they hold that lead to their different ways of looking at the problem?*
- *How would you see the main differences between what would happen to your child over the next year if he were treated as if he were delinquent or if he were treated as if she were ill?*

Juxtapositioning allows network members to consider in an uncensored way, the contrasting implications of extreme or amplified positions.

Mapping Out Emotions

Often competing or polarized factions emerge, with faction members locked into strong coalitions and yawning gulfs of animosity separating these subgroups. Typically, the professionals who adopt such polarized positions in child protection cases experience the strong emotional countertransference reactions described in Chapter 11. So, for example, in a physical child abuse case, inevitably there will be one faction of the professional network whose CTR is *rescuing the parents,* and this faction will polarise with those whose CTR is *rescuing the child.* In sexual abuse cases usually the faction whose CTR is *rescuing the father* polarize with those whose CTR is *rescuing the mother and child and persecuting the father* (Carr, 1989). Diagrams mapping out these polarized patterns, based on Karpman's triangle, are set out in Figures 15.6 and 15.7. Karpman's triangle has been described in Chapter 10.

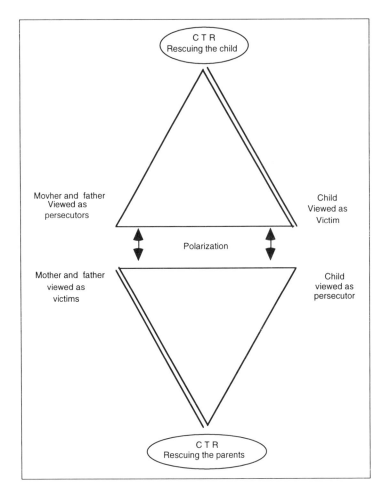

Figure 15.6. *Polarization of two countertransference reactions:*
rescuing the child and rescuing the parents

Mapping Out Alliances

Figures 15.6 and 15.7, which schematically describe polarizations of professionals with particular countertransference reactions, map onto the diamond-shaped diagrams of the symmetrical competitive system or the complimentary cooperative systems described by the fifth Province team and set out in Figures 15.8 and 15.9 (Colgan, 1991; McCarthy and Byrne, 1988). These figures schematically map out two common organizational structures families and involved statutory social workers adopt following the disclosure of sexual abuse. In the symmetrical competitive system, the abused daughter and the statutory social worker are aligned in a close relationship in symmetrical opposition to the mother and father who are also aligned in a close relationship. In this instance the parents deny the abuse and the social workers may find themselves experiencing the CTR of rescuing the child. In the complimentary cooperative system, the mother, daughter and statutory social worker become aligned in a cooperative way

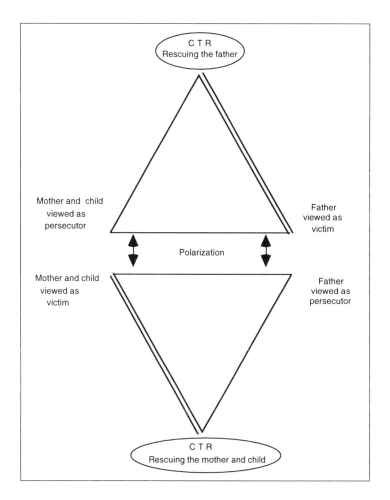

Figure 15.7. Polarization of two countertransference reactions: rescuing the father and rescuing the mother and daughter

and the father is excluded or blamed. Here the predominant CTR for the statutory worker is rescuing the mother and child.

The fifth Province team argue that workable solutions to problems cannot be found if therapists align themselves with any one point on these diamonds. Rather, the therapists must adopt a dis-position in the imaginal space at the centre of the diamond. From this neutral vantage point—this dis-position—they may explore the ambivalences within the system by questioning members of the system about the implications of maintaining extreme positions and exploring the differences between extreme positions. Questioning at the extremes and juxtapositioning, described earlier, are two of the key inquiry styles used. Incidentally, the fifth Province team, is so named because the dis-position it adopts at the imaginal centre of its diamonds reflects a mythical Irish province for its members. This province was an imaginal place where oppositions were resolved and unrelated things coincided (Hederman and Kearney, 1977).

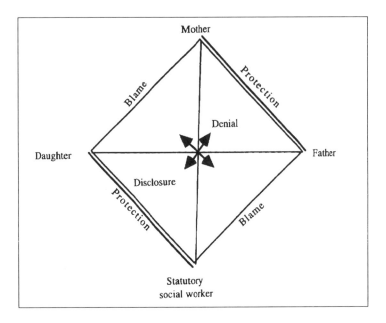

Figure 15.8.   Diamond map of the symmetrical competitive system which emerges following disclosure of father-daughter incest

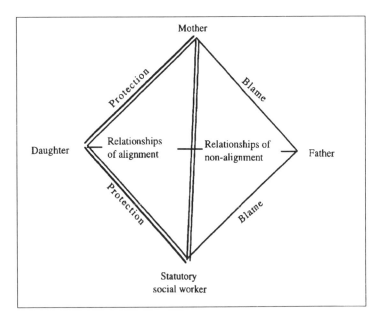

Figure 15.9.   Diamond map of the complementary co-operative system which emerges following disclosure of father-daughter incest

SUMMARY

Network meetings are convened when a therapeutic system is in a state of transition, crisis or extreme stuckness. When convening a network meeting set clear goals and make sure that the customer, the legal guardian and the involved social control agent attend, since little progress may be made without them. The goals of network meetings may be to clarify the customer and the contract, to construct a formulation, or to develop action plans. Open the meeting with introductions and set the agenda and the rules for participation clearly. Make sure that everyone gets a fair hearing by helping the reticent to elaborate their positions and the talkative condense their contributions. Summarize periodically to help members maintain focus. Above all, retain neutrality by siding with no one, curiously inquiring about each persons position and challenging each network member to develop an interactional framing of the problem and its resolution. Use time-out, if necessary, to integrate contribution into an interactional formulation and elaborate options for action. Once the meeting accepts the tentative integration, request a commitment to develop an action plan. Then work towards that by examining options.

In conflict ridden network meetings map out symmetrical or complimentary relationships between families and professionals, the ecology of ideas, the pattern of alliances, the major countertransference reactions of members, and use questioning at the extremes and juxtapositioning to break down the polarization process.

When contributing to a network meeting prepare points on your involvement, your hypotheses and plans. Use slack time to build working alliances. Always introduce yourself before making your first contribution. Outline your involvement first and hypotheses and plans later. Make your points briefly and summarize your points at the end of each major contribution. When you disagree, focus on clarifying the issue not on attacking the person with whom you disagree. Keep notes on who attended, on the formulation and on the plan If you have unresolved ambivalent feelings after the meeting, discuss these in supervision. You may find the methods for mapping out polarizations and alliance patterns useful in making sense of these mixed feelings.

Exercise 15.1.

Work as a single group.

Select a complex case where a number of professionals are involved and where there is currently a plausible reason for holding a network meeting.

The person who is working with the case must brief the rest of the group about it.

Decide which group members will play which roles in the exercise.

The convenor of the network meeting should then invite the network members to the meeting explaining the reason for it.

Family members should take about 10 minutes talking together agreeing in detail about how they are currently managing their problems and their daily routines and what they hope to get out of the network meeting.

Each person role-playing a professional should plan how they intend to contribute to the meeting.

The convenor should plan and conduct a network meeting following the guidelines set out in Figure 15.2.

Those role-playing professionals should follow the guidelines for contributing to network meetings set out in Figure 15.3.

Conduct a 30 minute network meeting.

Derole after the exercise.

Take 20 minutes to discuss
1.   The experience of family members in the meeting
2.   The areas in which the convenor and professionals contributing to the meeting felt competent and the areas in which they were challenged during the meeting.

Exercise 15.2.

Work in pairs.

Reflect on the case role-played in Exercise 15.1.

Using the conceptual mapping systems set out in the chapter, analyse the way the network was functioning in terms of

- Complimentary or symmetrical relationships
- Ecology of ideas
- Polarization of countertransference reactions
- Alliances and factions

As a single group discuss how these analyses might be useful in managing the case.

16

Disengagement

In Chapter 15, we left the Barrow Case as the network meeting ended. Let us rejoin Caroline, Dick and Sheila, a week later at the next family consultation and trace the progress of the Barrows through to the final session which occurred a month later. Mention will also be made of a follow-up phonecall which was made some months after this during the summer.

SESSION 6: HOLY THURSDAY

This session was divided into three thirty minute slots. first, Caroline was seen with her parents. Then she was seen alone and this was followed by a meeting with Sheila and Dick.

In the family review meeting, Caroline said that her pains had been intense but brief (eight on a ten point scale) for the Thursday and Friday following the network meeting. She had managed them herself by trying to distract herself with school work and by chatting to Kirsty during the break. On Friday morning, she sat outside class for five minutes, but found that she could handle the pain better if she went inside and participated in class. On Monday, Tuesday and Wednesday of the week leading up to the appointment, she had had only very brief episodes of pain of low intensity: about four on a ten point scale. She had missed no school.

In the individual session, Caroline said that she had begun to believe that the pain was a headache in her stomach. She said that she and Sheila had not fought in the mornings and that things at home were easier over the weekend. She went to a disco on the Saturday night; Dick had then driven her home and they had listened to a tape she had borrowed from a friend on the way. This was something completely new. Dick had never driven her home from a dance before or listened to her music.

Finally, in reviewing the network meeting, she said that it was a very difficult and embarrassing experience, but that in the end she felt like everyone finally listened to her and that things were turning out for the best.

This sentiment was echoed by Dick and Sheila, who said that they felt at first as if they were on trial for failing as parents. But that maybe it was worth it because Caroline had been different since. Sheila said that Dick had phoned her on a couple of occasions to check how things were going around breakfast time and that this had made it easier to avoid checking up on Caroline's health. Dick said that Sheila had been very understanding about his work situation and that Caroline had begun to take an interest in how his business worked. This surprised him.

A follow-up appointment was made for four weeks later.

SESSION 7: AFTER EASTER

The atmosphere in this session was celebratory. Caroline said that the pains had stopped completely over the Easter holidays and had not recurred. She had taken up yoga and was going to a modern dance class. She joked that while Dick had listened to her new tape a month ago, she knew that her music would never be to his taste. She and Dick had engaged in some normal teenage fights about loud music over the preceding month. They both joked about this, particularly when Sheila asked Dick to try to be more understanding.

Sheila and Dick were planning a spring vacation together in the Lake District. They had not been away together as a couple since Mat's birth, eighteen years previously. So they were looking forward to this with joy and excitement. Caroline was going to stay over at Kirsty's while her parents were away.

The heart of the session focused on beliefs about the permanence of the change and on relapse management. All three family members did not believe that the changes were a transitory *flash in the pan*. They saw them as permanent. This, they said, was because they saw the changes as part of a wider change in the patterns of interaction within the family. They identified that the cycle of interaction around the presenting problem had been disrupted by Sheila agreeing not to ask Caroline about her health in the morning; by Dick spontaneously phoning Sheila occasionally to check if she was coping, and by Caroline taking responsibility for managing the pain if it occurred at school. They also noted that Caroline felt more connected to Dick. In the past she had felt threatened by him. It was also apparent to them, that Sheila and Dick's relationship was now stronger and more supportive. finally, they noted that the involvement of the professional network in their family life had virtually ceased, and that this allowed them to get on with day to day activities as opposed to worrying about the problem. All of these things appeared to be stable and enduring. Taken together, these changes suggested to the Barrows that Caroline's pains and school non-attendance were a thing of the past.

I said then, in keeping with the humorous atmosphere in the session, that I had good news and bad news. The good news was that the changes were probably permanent. The bad news was that relapses were inevitable. I explained that if the family underwent stress related to Mat going to college, Dick having work hassles, Caroline having problems with school or boyfriends, or Sheila having difficulties of any sort, I would not be surprised if the morning fights recurred, Caroline's pains began again, and a split between Dick and Sheila about how to manage them recurred. This, I explained, happens with all bad habits. Problem drinkers and ex-smokers often relapse under stress. But, I suggested that if they simply repeated the solution that they used had on this occasion to handle the problem the relapse would be very brief. If need be they could call me and request a booster session. During this discussion, the occurrence of relapses under stress was related to the three column formulation.

Throughout this monologue, Caroline appeared to be very edgy. I suspected that this might reflect her anxiety about relapsing but I was wrong. Her main concern was to leave the session early so that she could get to her dance class on time at 5.30pm. This reticence about therapy is common in the later stages. Once problems have been solved, most youngsters just want to get on with life! She left in a hurry.

In the final thirty minutes of the session, Dick and Sheila talked openly about the strain that Dick's work and Sheila's bereavement had placed on their marriage and how they had found it increasingly difficult to talk openly to each other. They noticed that this had begun to change since the network meeting. They hoped that this change would continue. I offered them the option of coming for a couple of sessions at some point in the future, without Caroline, to discuss the marital issues that they had raised. They said that they might take me up on the offer but they never did.

FOLLOW-UP PHONECALL

Four months later, in August, I called to see how the Barrows were getting along and spoke to Sheila and Caroline. The family had experienced a relapse in mid-June following a major row between Dick and Mat about college. However, Dick and Sheila had spoken to Caroline about it and said that she should take her time and be patient and the pains would go away. Dick phoned Sheila regularly each morning during this period and so Sheila was in a position to support Caroline. As to the row about college: Dick and Mat eventually resolved their differences and Mat was due to leave for university in October.

Sheila and Dick had enjoyed their Spring Break in the Lake District immensely, and planned to take vacations away together more often. This was my final contact with the Barrow family. A summary of the case is set out in Figure 16.1.

The final sessions with the Barrows and the follow-up phonecall highlight a number of important points about the disengagement process which will serve as the focus for this chapter.

SIX DISENGAGEMENT/RECONTRACTING SITUATIONS

In Positive Practice, disengagement is primarily related to the therapeutic contract. In Chapter 1 and Figure 1.1 it was noted that disengagement is a distinct therapeutic phase where goal attainment is reviewed. The goals and the number of sessions are both agreed following the construction of a three column formulation. In Positive Practice a distinction is made between the following disengagement/recontracting situations.

1. Situations where goal attainment occurs before the end of the series of sessions agreed in the initial contract.

Timing	Session structure	Pain	School Attendance
Session 1 12.2.90 Monday 10am 3 days after referral letter	Contract for assessment agreed Assessment completed Presentation of formulation Contract for treatment agreed Caroline given pain monitoring task Sheila and Dick given options discussion task	7	60%
Session 2 23.2.90 Friday 5pm A week after session 1	Tasks completed Goal set Pain management training occurs in the session	5	78%
Session 3 8.3.90 Thursday 7pm A fortnight after session 2	Tasks completed Communication and problem solving training for Sheila and Dick in the session	5	67%
Session 4 22.3.90 Thursday 2pm A fortnight after session 3	Dick absent from session Tasks incomplete Statement of dilemma Letter to Dick	6	60%
Crisis phonecall 2.4.90 Monday 10am 10 days after session 4 Five days before next scheduled appointment	Dick drove Caroline to school and she would not leave the car Dick phoned to request individual psychiatric evaluation	8	57%
Session 5 4.4.90 Wednesday 4pm 2 days after crisis phonecall	Caroline gives her account in an individual session Sheila, Dick, Caroline, teacher, school nurse and GP attend a network meeting Plan for school reentry and pain management developed	8	0%
Session 6 12.4.90 Thursday 7pm A week after Network meeting on Holy Thursday	Session divided into 3, 30 minute slots Family review Caroline's individual slot Sheila and Dick's parental slot	8 for Mon Tues Wed then 4	100%
Session 7 11.5 .90 Friday 4pm A month after session 6 Back at school 2 weeks since end of Easter holidays	Session divided into two slots Family review Sheila and Dick's parental slot	2	100%
Follow up phonecall 3.8.90 Friday 11am Three months after session 7	Talked to Sheila and Caroline	0	100%

Figure 16.1.   Summary of consultation process with the Barrow family

2. Situations where goal attainment occurs at the end of the end of the series of sessions agreed in the initial contract.
3. Situations where partial goal attainment is noted at the end of the series of sessions agreed in the initial contract but where it is clear that this improvement may not be sustained without further therapy.
4. Situations where, at the end of the series of sessions agreed in the initial contract, goal attainment occurs but where it is clear that further consultation focusing on child problems, marital problems or individual therapy may be requested.
5. Situations where no progress has been made or where deterioration has occurred.
6. Situations where families drop out of treatment.

In situations 1 and 2 with cases where the consultation process has been effective at or before the number of sessions in the original contract have been completed, disengagement is relatively easy. For example, with the Barrows the goals (described in Chapter 8) were achieved within the agreed limit of six sessions (described in Chapter 7) following the intake interview. The disengagement process only required spacing the therapy sessions further apart, focusing on relapse prevention and leaving open the possibility of occasional consultation or booster sessions as required. In situations 3 and 4, recontracting for further work is the central task therapeutic task. In situations 5 and 6, analysing the reasons for lack of progress, deterioration or dropout, and liaising with the referring agent are the central therapeutic responsibilities. Let us look at each of these disengagement skills in detail.

PHASING OUT THERAPY

With the Barrows, a period of a month separated the penultimate and final sessions, whereas previous sessions were separated by no more than two weeks. This was an intentional phasing out of therapy. Sometimes the phasing out may be spread across a number of sessions (Heath, 1985). The Milan group were among the first to suggest that less time-intensive therapy may be more effective (Selvini-Palazzoli, 1980). They argued that a longer interval between sessions allowed the family system time to respond to interventions. This idea may usefully be applied to the disengagement process. In Positive Practice, once progress begins, schedule sessions further apart. This sends clients the message that you are developing confidence in their ability to manage their difficulties without sustained professional help. A crucial part of spacing sessions further apart is framing the process in a way that helps the family develop a sense of competence (rather than a sense of rejection). Here are some examples of how increasing the inter-session interval may be framed so as to promote positive change.

- *From what you've said today it sounds like things are beginning to improve. It would be useful to know how you would sustain this sort of improvement over a period longer than a fortnight. So lets leave the gap between this session and the next a bit longer, say three weeks or a month?*
- *It seems that you've got a way of handling this thing fairly independently now. I suggest that we meet again in a month, rather than a week, and then discuss how you went about managing things independently over a four week period. How does that sound to you?*

BELIEFS ABOUT THE PERMANENCE OF CHANGE

In the final session with the Barrows, I inquired about the Barrows understanding of the major improvement that Caroline showed by asking the following question:

• *Do you think that Caroline's improvement is a permanent thing or just a flash in the pan?*

This sort of question is useful to ask during the disengagement process where some degree of goal attainment has occurred. It throws light on the way in which family members construe the changes that have occurred. If the change is seen as transitory, then it is important to inquire what additional events would have to occur in order for change to be construed as relatively enduring. That is, the following sorts of questions would need to be asked:

• *How would you know if the improvement was not just a flash in the pan?*
• *What do you think your dad/mum/wife/ husband/ would have to see happening in order to be convinced that these changes were here to stay?*

The answers to these sorts of questions will suggest interventions that may help family members come to construe improvement as relatively permanent. For example, the father of a sixteen year old boy who was referred because he had stolen money at home and repeatedly got drunk, said that he would know his son's improvement was permanent, when three months had gone by without incident and when the boy did some work around the house without being asked. Three further sessions were scheduled at monthly intervals. The father was asked to keep a daily diary of any signs of spontaneous help on the son's part. The diary was reviewed in the sessions. In the second of these the father confessed that he had gathered sufficient evidence of spontaneous help on his son's part to be convinced that the change was permanent.

Once family members are convinced that relatively enduring change has occurred, it is useful to ask for their theory about why they believe it is permanent rather than transitory. This will help them recap how symptomatic relief is related to systemic change through reference to the three column formulation of their problems. This process of recapping the relationship between the symptom, the problem-system and the therapeutic system is a central part of termination in the McMaster model of family therapy (Epstein and Bishop, 1981).

RELAPSE MANAGEMENT

Because empirical evidence suggests that with child and family psychological problems relapses are very common, relapse management is a critical part of Positive Practice (Herbert, 1991). When clients show that they believe enduring change has occurred, and when they have recapped the way in which they found a solution to their presenting problems, they are in a position to consider the relapse management process. The therapist's task is to help clients develop a framework for predicting the conditions under which relapse may occur and then constructing a plan for their management. However, the process begins by introducing the idea of relapse in as manageable a way as possible. Here is an example of how this may be done in a case where Barry, the son, successfully learned from his father, Danny, how to manage explosive temper tantrums. The following excerpt is addressed to Barry's mother.

- *You said to me that you are convinced now that Barry has control over his temper......that he has served an apprenticeship to his Dad in learning how to manage this fierce anger that he sometimes feels. OK....? It looks like the change is here to stay also... that's what you believe. That's what I believe. But there may be some exceptions to this rule. Maybe on certain occasions he may slip....and have a big tantrum....Like when you gave up cigarettes, Danny, and then had one at Christmas in the pub......a relapse....It may be that Barry will have a temper relapse. Lets talk about how to handle relapses?*

Many relatively simple behavioural problems may be used as analogies to introduce the idea of relapse. Smoking, drinking, nail-biting, thumb-sucking, and accidentally sleeping late in the morning are among some of the more useful options to consider. It is crucial that key members of the family understand the analogy. Parents find it easy to empathize with the idea of a child relapsing if they themselves have been heavy smokers, quit and later relapsed. Siblings will easily identify with habits like nail biting, thumb-sucking or sleeping late. Once all family members have accepted the concept of relapse, then the therapist asks how such events might be predicted or anticipated.

- *If that were going to happen in what sort of situations do you think it would be most likely to occur?*
- *What signs would you look for, if you were going to predict a relapse?*
- *From what you know about the way the problem started this time, how would you be able to tell that a relapse was about to happen?*

Often relapses are triggered by similar factors to those that precipitated the original problem. For example, Lucinda, a nine year old pianist, began refusing food shortly before a major concert. About eighteen months later she relapsed before another major performance. Sometimes relapses occur as an anniversary reaction. This is often the case in situations where a loss has occurred and where the loss or the bereavement precipitated the original referral. More generally, relapses seem to be associated with a build up of stressful life events (Cummings, Gordon and Marlatt, 1980). These factors include family transitions such as members leaving or joining the family system; family transformation through divorce or remarriage; family illness; changes in children's school situation; changes in parents' work situation; or changes in the financial status of the family. finally, relapses may be associated with the interaction between physical environmental factors and constitutional vulnerabilities. For example, people diagnosed as having seasonal affective disorder are particularly prone to relapse in early winter (Wehr and Rosenthal, 1989), and youngsters with asthma may be prone to relapse in the spring (Lask and Matthew, 1979).

Once family members have considered events that might precipitate a relapse, inquire about the way in which these events will be translated into a full-blown relapse.

- *Sometimes when a relapse occurs, people do things without thinking and this makes things worse. Like with cigarettes...... if you nag someone that has relapsed, they will probably smoke more to deal with the hassle of being nagged!! Just say a relapse happened with Barry, what would each of you do ....if you acted without thinking......that would make things worse?*

This type of inquiry allows family members an opportunity to apply the framework they constructed in the three column formulation of the original problem to a new but similar situation. This is often a very humorous part of the consultation process, where the therapist can encourage clients to exaggerate what they believe their own and other family members automatic reactions would be and how these would lead to an escalation of the problem. The final set of inquiries about relapse management focus on the family's plans for handling the relapse. Here are some examples.

- *Just say a relapse happened, what do you think each person in the family should do?*
- *You found a solution to the problem this time round. Say a relapse happened, how would you use the same solution again?*

In Positive Practice, the therapist's role is to acknowledge that the family, at this stage of the consultation process, has most (if not all) of the answers. Where families have made substantial progress towards stated goals, they will usually develop useful relapse management plans. If the therapist has anything to add to the refinement of relapse management plans, suggestions should be offered as minor modifications rather than major revisions. This supports rather than undermines families' confidence in their own problem-solving abilities.

DISENGAGEMENT AS PART OF A RELATIONSHIP

If long term therapy runs the risk of fostering client dependency, brief approaches to consultation, like Positive Practice, may leave families feeling abandoned. Providing clients with a way of construing disengagement as the end of an episode of contact rather than as the end of a relationship is a useful way of avoiding engendering feelings of abandonment. Three strategies may be used to achieve this. first, a distant follow-up appointment may be scheduled. Second, families may be told that they have *a session in the bank* which they can make use of whenever they need it without having to take their turn on the waiting list again. Third, telephone back-up may be offered to help the family manage relapses. In all three instances, families may disengage from the regular process of consultations, while at the same time remaining connected to the therapeutic system.

With families where there are chronic problems, construing the disengagement as marking the end of an episode rather than the end of a relationship is particularly important. I am referring here to families where a member has a chronic illness, a physical disability or a mental handicap. I am also referring to multiproblem families with multiagency involvement, such as those where child protection is an ongoing concern. In these cases, each time a therapy contract is completed, the family and involved professionals are invited to recontact the therapist as further problems arise or at critical transitions in the family lifecycle. In this way, Positive Practice provides a framework for long term involvement while retaining a brief-therapy approach to consultation.

HANDING OVER

Where clinical psychology trainees, junior medical doctors on rotation, locum therapists or other transient staff are closing cases where goal attainment has occurred and the therapy contract has been completed, it is good for both the client and the agency for a permanent staff member to be invited into a portion of the final session. This allows the departing clients to identify the permanent staff member with their therapist and the clinic. In Positive Practice, the therapist who has worked with the family uses the handover period to introduce the family to the permanent staff member. This is also an excellent opportunity to frame problem resolution as reflecting the family's strengths. Here is an example of a former colleague handing over a case that included a single mother, Alice, and her three children, Roz, Penny and Sam.

- *Alice, Roz. Penny.....and Sam..this is Alan Carr, Clinical Psychologist at the unit. I said to you earlier that I am leaving the clinic ....shortly. Anyway....I wanted you to meet Alan who will be available to you as a h...a sounding board if you need a further meeting. Let me fill you in on where we've got to......(to AC)...A big concern was this....fighting about family rules. Most of the work that has been done has focused on agreeing a set of rules and finding a way to cut back on fighting time and increase fun time. Sam, Roz, Penny and Alice have worked really hard on that one and put together a list of house rules that they are working with right now. Roz...she is six now....she came to the clinic with a big problem. Didn't you (to Roz)... You wanted to learn how to use the toilet properly like a big girl. Well, you have learned now. Let us all look at your star chart for this last week seven gold stars. Isn't that wonderful. And you did this week all by yourself. ....Alice has stuck with the programme through thick and thin over about six weeks...even when the going got rough she stuck with it. We have talked about getting control of the bladder as a developmental problem and the star chart training programme as a way for Alice to help Roz develop....That's about it.........*

When handing over a case let clients know that you are handing over to a colleague whom you respect and trust at a professional level. Let them see that you value their strengths and problem solving skills. finally let them see that the role offered to the colleague to whom you are handing over fits with the family's current need. In the example just given the need was for a sounding board. In a crisis, the need might be for a colleague to offer advice on crisis management.

RECONTRACTING AND REFERRING ON

In the final session with the Barrows, when Caroline had left, Sheila and Dick spontaneously brought up a marital issue which was a major concern for both of them. The issue was the effect of Dick's work on the quality of the marital relationship and on family life. An offer of a contract for further consultations in this area was made. The other issue for which a further contract could have been offered was Sheila's unresolved grief related to both her mother's death and to the miscarriage.

In my experience, in virtually all families that are referred with child-focused problems, both marital and individual adult issues that could serve as a potential focus for further consultation emerge. In Positive Practice these are acknowledged, but offering a contract for consultation or referral to another agency to deal with them is usually deferred until the child-focused problem has been dealt with, unless there is good reason not to wait.

The reasoning behind this approach is as follows. first, if family and therapist devote their energy to solving more than one problem at a time, then the chance of failure increases because of the increased demands on the family's coping resources. Second, if families successfully solve a child-focused problem, this may enhance their view of themselves as good problem solvers. Therapy may then progress to dealing effectively with marital and adult issues without the help of a therapist. Third, and most importantly, the original therapeutic contract is to focus on a child-centred problem. The therapist therefore has no mandate to address marital or adult individual problems without very good reason. If the therapist, without an agreed contract, begins to explore marital or adult individual issues in a family session, the parents may find this invasive or threatening and drop out of therapy.

For example, the parents of a teenage boy referred because he ran away from home appeared to have serious marital problems. The family dropped out of treatment after two sessions. Later feedback from the family doctor confirmed that they dropped out because they felt as if too much of the consultation time was focusing on their relationship and not enough time was being devoted to parenting issues.

The main exceptions to the rule of deferring marital and adult issues until the contract for child-focused problems is completed, are those situations which are dangerous or which seriously compromise the parents problem solving abilities. Marital violence, self-injurious behaviour, clinical depression and psychotic symptoms are among the most common examples of such problems. In each of these instances, in Positive Practice, the therapist points out that the child-focused work cannot progress until the outstanding marital or individual adult issue is dealt with.

DISENGAGEMENT

1.   Increase the intersession interval when improvement begins
2.   Review goal attainment when the session contract is complete or before it if improvement is obvious
3.   If goals are not reached, do not do *more of the same*
4.   If goals have been achieved, find out if the family believe the change is temporary or permanent
5.   Help the family construct an understanding of the change process
6.   Discuss relapse management
7.   Construct disengagement as an episodic event rather than as the end of a relationship
8.   Schedule follow-up.

Figure 16.2.   Guidelines for disengagement

Here is an example of a contract for marital work being offered to a violent couple who originally came to the clinic because their son was encopretic.

- *The main problem you wanted help with....when you first came ... was Mike's soiling. And we agreed to work on that....I thought I could help you with that one. But now I know that I can't....You see.......the way you describe things....with the fighting and the hitting at home....that even if you follow through on trying to manage Mike differently ...he will still soil. He soils when he sees mum and dad hitting each other..But we have no agreement to discuss this issue... the violence..the hitting. This is true? But I am willing to discuss an agreement with you now, if you would like that. This agreement is a marital issue. So if you want to discuss it with me I suggest we deal with this without Mike and the girls? Just take a minute to think about that now and tell me if this is something you want or not?*

Ethical dilemmas posed in cases of marital violence are discussed in Chapter 17. Guidelines for disengagement are summarized in Figure 16.2.

LACK OF GOAL ATTAINMENT, DETERIORATION AND DROPOUT

In some cases if clear progress towards the therapeutic goals set at the outset of the consultation process is being made, a further contract for a limited number of extra sessions may be made. A major pitfall in Positive Practice, however, is to continue the consultation process indefinitely without a review of progress towards goals and without a clear session limit to the therapeutic contract. This type of open-ended therapy can lead to the therapist and clients developing a pattern of interaction which maintains rather than resolves the problem.

In cases where no progress toward goals has been made at the end of a time limited period such as sic or twelve sessions, then the clients and the therapist must accept that the approach to therapy described here is not suitable for the problems presented, and referral back to the original referring agent or on to another professional, agency or treatment modality with the consent of the referring agent may be considered. In other instances clients drop out of therapy. In about 10% of cases families deteriorate as a result of therapy (Carr, 1991a).

Where dropout, deterioration or lack of goal attainment occurs, a crucial aspect of Positive Practice is analysing why this occurred. In Coleman's (1985) *Failures in Family Therapy* leading family therapists offer detailed analyses of their own therapeutic failures, and these cases serve as useful models for all clinicians who want to understand why, in some instances, therapy does not help.

Failures may occur for a number of reasons. first, they may occur because of the engagement difficulties described in Chapter 2. The correct members of the problem-system may not have been engaged. For example, if the customer is not engaged, dropout is inevitable. The construction of a three column formulation which does not open up possibilities for change is a second possible reason for failure. A third reason why failure occurs may be that the therapist did not design therapeutic tasks appropriately, or had difficulties in offering the family invitations to complete the therapeutic tasks. Problems with handling families' reservations about change, and the apparent resistance that this gives rise to, is a fourth and further source of failure. A fifth possible cause of failure is the mismanagement of therapeutic crises and accommodating to families' demands that the therapist abandon an interactional problem formulation in favour of an individualistic formulation. Disengaging without empowering the family to handle relapses is a sixth possible factor contributing to therapeutic failure. A seventh factor is countertransference. Where countertransference reactions seriously compromise therapist neutrality and the capacity to join in an empathic way with each member of the problem-system therapeutic failure may occur.

Finally, failure may occur because the goals set did not take account of the constraints within which family members were operating. These constraints include biological factors such as illness, psychological factors such as mental handicap, economic factors such as poverty, social factors such as general life stress, and broader socio-cultural factors such as minority group membership.

The analysis of treatment failure is an important way to develop therapeutic skill. A checklist for analysing treatment failure is contained in Figure 16.3.

FAILURE ANALYSIS

1. Engagement problems
2. Formulation did not open up possibilities
3. Tasks poorly designed or offered
4. Problems with managing resistance and beliefs about change
5. Accommodating to individualistic problem formulation in a crisis
6. Inadequate preparation for relapse
7. Violation of neutrality
8. Set goals without taking constraints into account
   (biological/psychological/economic/social/cultural)

Figure 16.3.   A checklist for failure analysis

LOSS

Disengagement often leads to a sense of loss. Where therapy has been unsuccessful, disengagement may lead to a sense of loss of professional expertise. Loss of an important source of professional affirmation and friendship are often experienced when therapists disengage from successful cases. Let us look at both types of loss in more detail.

Where therapists attribute many therapy failures to their own personal or professional inadequacy, they lose their sense of personal and professional self-worth. This loss in turn may lead at an emotional level to sadness that one has not met personal expectations, anger that clients have caused this, and anxiety that the process of repeated failure may continue. At a cognitive level it may lead therapists to believe that there is nothing that they can do to be effective in helping clients. At a behavioural level it may lead to an avoidance of clinical work and a retreat into other activities such as administration or participation in fruitless professional meetings. At a somatic level it may lead to frequent illness due to immunological deficiencies associated with the stress of repeated failure. This analysis is based on my own clinical experience, on the burnout literature (Malasch, 1982), on the learned helplessness model of depression (Abramson, Seligman and Teasdale, 1978) and on recent advances in psychoneuroimmunology (Levy and Heiden, 1991). The key to managing therapeutic failure is first to analyse all failures using the framework outlined above so that you can understand intellectually the precise factors that contributed to the lack of goal attainment. Second, and most important, is to examine the analysis of failed cases within a supervision context with peers or more experienced clinicians. The supervision context provides the technical and emotional support required to understand unsuccessful cases and work through emotional reactions to them.

Disengagement from successful cases may also lead to a profound sense of loss, since such cases when they are ongoing may affirm both the personal and professional identify of the therapist. At an emotional level, the actual or expected loss may be experienced as both sadness and anger: sadness that clients who affirmed your identity have gone or will leave, and anger that despite your attachment to them, they have abandoned you or are about to so. At a behavioural level, anticipated disengagement in successful cases may lead therapists to prolong the consultation process unnecessarily or to disengage too abruptly. After disengagement in successful cases the sense of loss may lead to anger towards new clients or to an avoidance of them. Underpinning this may be a belief that no new client can take the place of the successful clients from whom you have recently disengaged. Overly abrupt endings, prolonged consultation, avoidance of new clients, and related feelings of anger and sadness are all issues requiring analysis and discussion in supervision with peers or experienced clinicians.

Fortunately, much of the time, therapists are not overwhelmed by the disengagement process and manage it satisfactorily.

PROBLEMS WITH STRATEGIC DISENGAGEMENT

Strategic therapists argue that, in certain resistant cases, the therapist may tell clients that further therapy is no longer necessary and frame this in such a way that clients are forced to solve their own problems (Weeks and L'Abate, 1982). In other instances strategic therapists interpret dropout as indicating that therapy has been successful. Clients who drop out are assumed to have found a way to cope with their problems without the help of a therapist. With strategic disengagement or a strategic interpretation of dropout, clients are usually unaware that the therapist assumes that the paradoxical position he or she has taken has led to their improvement. There are a number of problems with this viewpoint (Treacher, 1989). The most obvious is that the strategic position provides no opportunity for the client to negotiate the disengagement process. The second problem is that the strategic stance provides no avenue through which the therapist can obtain feedback from the client on therapeutic effectiveness in the from follow-up data. In Positive Practice, strategic approaches to disengagement are avoided unless no viable alternative is available.

SUMMARY

The process of disengagement begins once improvement is noticed. The interval between sessions is increased at this point. The degree to which goals have been met is reviewed when the session contract is complete or before this, if improvement is obvious. If goals have been achieved, the family's beliefs about the permanence of this change is established. Then the therapist helps the family construct an understanding of the change process. Relapse management is discussed and the way in which stress can trigger the processes described in the three column formulation is highlighted. Disengagement is constructed as an episodic event rather than as the end of a relationship. This is particularly important when working with families where members have chronic problems. In some instances, the end of one therapeutic contract will lead immediately to the beginning of a further contract. This subsequent contract may focus on the original child centred problems, marital difficulties, or individual work for the adults in the family. Referral to other therapists or agencies for this further work may be appropriate.

In Positive Practice, if goals are not reached, the therapist avoids doing *more of the same* (Segal, 1991). Rather, therapeutic failures are analysed in a systematic way. The understanding that emerges from this is useful both for the clients and for the therapist. From the clients' perspective, they avoid becoming trapped in a consultation process that maintains rather than resolves the problem. From the therapists' viewpoint it provides a mechanism for coping with burnout that occurs when multiple therapeutic failures occur.

Exercise 16.1.

This exercise is based on the White case first mentioned in Exercise 13.2. Reread the referral letter, the piece about the therapeutic crisis and the formulation.

In this exercise the family have reached their goals. Karen has now maintained her weight for 6 months, although there have been times when her weight has dropped significantly for a couple of weeks. There have been six monthly sessions.

Divide the training group into members who will role-play the family and members who will act as therapist and team.

Family members should take about 10 minutes talking together agreeing in detail about how they have managed the previous six months.

The therapist and team should use this time to plan how they will manage a disengagement interview with the Whites.

The therapist must then conduct a 30 minute session following the guidelines for disengagement described in Figure 16.2.

Derole after the exercise.

Take 20 minutes to discuss
1.   The family's experience during the disengagement interview
2.   The areas in which the therapist felt competent and the areas in which the therapist felt challenged when managing the disengagement interview.

Exercise 16.2.

Work in pairs.

Select a case where therapeutic failure occurred.

Analyse it using the guidelines set out in Figure 16.3.

Write down the main points that you believe led to failure.

Discuss these together as a group.

17

Ethical Issues

We make ethical judgements in every clinical consultation. Many of these judgements are made intuitively without extensive conscious critical evaluation. For example, the practice of adopting a position of neutrality, at an ethical level, is a judgement to give all members of the system a fair hearing. Once the skill of adopting a position of neutrality has been developed, it becomes an automatic way of dealing with the ethical problem of fairness and equity in family consultations. Intuitive ethical judgements are based not only on clinical techniques (such as neutrality) derived from theoretical models (such as systemic consultation), but also on personal ethical principles, professional codes of ethics and the sociolegal context within which the consultation occurs. With experience, the range of ethical problems that can be dealt with at an intuitive level increases. An important factor contributing to the development of ethical intuition is the conscious critical evaluation and resolution of ethical dilemmas that have not been previously encountered by the clinician. In this chapter we will explore the management of ethical dilemmas.

An ethical dilemma is a situation where there is a conflict between two obligations, values or principles. Usually, each of the available courses of action appear to entail negative outcomes for some member of the problem-system. In working with children and their families, a number of situations commonly pose ethical dilemmas for clinicians. These include cases where child abuse and marital violence are suspected or have occurred. Cases where secrets are divulged to the therapist, or where it appears that paradoxical interventions may be particularly helpful to the family, also pose ethical dilemmas. Each of these situations will be discussed below.

FIVE FACTORS THAT INFORM ETHICAL DECISION MAKING

Before considering each of these situations, factors that inform ethical decision making will be considered. These include the practitioner's clinical model, their professional codes of ethics, the sociolegal context in which they work, their personal ethical principles and ethical theory (Woody, 1990; Zygmond and Boorhem, 1989).

Clinical Models

All clinical models entail prescriptions for the most fruitful course of action. Different models prescribe different courses of action. For example, in using Positive Practice as a clinical model with the Barrow case, Caroline's school non-attendance was construed as an interactional phenomenon requiring systemic consultation. It would have been unethical, from the point of view of Positive Practice, to accept an individualistic construction of Caroline's difficulties and their resolution. Were a psychoanalytic model used, the clinician would have engaged Caroline in individual therapy from the outset and focused on the analysis of defences and the interpretation of transference. From a psychoanalytic perspective, it would be unethical to include parents in the analytic sessions.

Not least because of their conflicting prescriptions, clinical models cannot be the sole basis for ethical decision making. However, in choosing between clinical models, those that have been shown in empirical outcome studies to be effective may offer a sounder basis for ethical decision making than those based on clinical insights alone.

Professional Ethical Codes

Professional codes of ethics are lists of rules or ethical prescriptions drawn up by representative bodies such as the Psychological Society of Ireland, the American Association of Marital and Family Therapy, or the British Psychological Society. A problem with such codes is that professionals may be members of two bodies that have different rules about issues such as client confidentiality, CPD, intimacy with ex-clients and so forth. Ethical decision cannot therefore be based only on professional codes of ethics.

The Sociolegal Context

The social, legal and organizational contexts within which a therapist works entail values which inform professionals' ethical decisions. These values are not static and evolve with changes in society, legislation and social policy. At a social level, for example, the AIDS crisis has generated a situation where now unprotected promiscuous sex in adolescence may be seen as a life threatening and ethically undesirable behaviour. This would not have been the case in the 1960s. At a legal level, the mandatory reporting of child abuse and the requirement, following the Tarasoff decision in the USA, that clinicians inform third parties of threats to their well-being made by their patients (Fulero, 1988), are examples of ethically prescribed courses of action that have evolved as laws have changed. At an organizational level, therapists have an ethical duty to fulfil their employment contracts, many of which are informed by social policy.

Often ethical prescriptions entailed by the sociolegal context may conflict with the best interest of a particular family. For example, in social service departments, workers may be unable to offer therapy to families in need because of a high case load and an agency policy to give priority to cases requiring child-protection-assessments. While sociolegal considerations, like clinical models and codes of ethics, inform ethical decision making; personal ethical principles and ethical theories also have a critical role to play.

Personal Ethical Principles

Personal ethical principles that inform ethical decision making are unique to each clinician. However, five principles of particular relevance to clinical practice are commonly held by many clinicians (Zygmond and Boorhem, 1989). The first of these, the principle of autonomy, entails a commitment to upholding clients' freedom of thought and action provided this does not interfere with the rights of others. The second principle of nonmaleficence is encapsulated in the Hippocratic oath: Do no harm. The corollary of this, the principle of beneficence, advocates a commitment to clients' health and welfare. Fidelity, the fourth principle, involves being trustworthy, respecting client confidentiality and privacy. Justice is the fifth principle. This entails a commitment to fairness, while taking account of the different needs, abilities and vulnerabilities of members of problem-systems. Ethical principles as a basis for ethical decision making are not without their shortcomings. At a personal level, therapists' religion, minority or majority group membership, personal philosophy, degree of training, and level of burnout may compromise their sense of fairness and commitment to the principle of justice in practice. Also, in some instances, ethical principles do not provide a clear guide to ethical decision making. For example, in cases of threatened self-injury, the principle of autonomy requires the therapist to respect the clients freedom to act, while the principle of beneficience demands that the therapist protect the client's welfare.

Ethical Theory

When ethical principles are in conflict, ethical theory may be used to decide which is the best course of action to take. Theories of ethics posit logical rules for making ethical decisions. Zygmond and Boorhem (1989) advocate the use of two particular ethical theories: universalizability and balancing theory. With universalizability, an ethical decision is one that can be generalized to all similar cases. With balancing theory, an ethical decision is one that entails the least amount of avoidable harm to all individuals even if this limits the benefits to those involved. Woody (1990) favours utilitarianism. Here, the most ethical course of action is that which leads to the greatest good for the greatest number. It is important to note that different ethical theories may point to different solutions to the same ethical dilemma.

Ethical Decision Making

When faced with an ethical dilemma, in Positive Practice, the clinician first identifies available courses of action. Then, the ethical status of each course of action may be evaluated with reference to clinical models, professional codes of ethics, sociolegal contextual factors, personal ethical principles and ethical theories. In the light of this analysis, an informed ethical judgement may be made. Let us turn now to areas in child and family practice that commonly pose ethical dilemmas for clinicians.

CHILD ABUSE

Intrafamilial child abuse is a complex phenomenon (Cicchetti and Carlson, 1989). Distinctions are made between physical, sexual and emotional child abuse as well as between child abuse and neglect. Distinctions may also be made between cases referred for other problems in which the consultation process leads the therapist to suspect the occurrence of child abuse and cases referred explicitly for either validation or rehabilitation. In all types of cases, there is a conflict between the need of the child for protection and safety and the desire of the parents to retain custody of the child.

In cases of suspected child abuse at the clinical level, one dilemma is whether to maintain neutrality and risk the danger of child abuse or abandon neutrality in favour of child protection. Lang, Little and Cronen (1990) distinguish between the domains of explanation, production and aesthetics. They argue that therapeutic neutrality is an appropriate position to adopt when working within the domain of explanations: the domain within which therapy is usually conducted. Within the domain of production, the domain within which child protection procedures are carried out, neutrality is an inappropriate position to adopt. The decision about which domain to operate in, they argue, is made within the domain of aesthetics and is informed by ethics and a commitment to elegant practice.

In cases of suspected child abuse, there are a number of dilemmas at a sociolegal level. There is a conflict between the obligation to the state to protect the child and an obligation to the family to maintain confidentiality. If the therapist invokes statutory powers to protect the child, then he or she is violating confidentiality. If the therapist does not take steps to protect the child, then the obligation to the state and the needs of the child are violated. If the therapist reports a suspected case of child abuse and there is insufficient evidence to support the suspicion, the child may be further endangered because the family may completely isolate itself from all helping agencies.

In cases where child abuse is validated, from the viewpoint of ethical balance theory, the impact of child protection proceedings, removal of the child from the family, or removal of the aggressor from the family, needs to be compared with the impact of leaving the child within the family where the abuse is occurring.

Within Positive Practice, the protection of the child is the priority. Therapy cannot proceed until a formulation which takes account of the abuse has been constructed and accepted by members of the family and the wider system. The construction of such a formulation may take many sessions where family and network members are seen individually and collectively. The therapist should carefully plan the assessment process, if child abuse is suspected, so that it maximizes the chance of securing a statutory order to protect the child if need be. In many cases this may involve arranging for a paediatric evaluation of a child's injuries, bruises or overall health in conjunction with a child protection worker. In cases of suspected sexual abuse it will involve arranging a videotaped interview between the child and a validation team (often a social worker and police officer). A major impediment to the construction of a formulation is the process of denial which often permeates the system. With all forms of abuse, invariably the abuser denies responsibility. In child sexual abuse the characteristic pattern is for disclosure by the victim to be followed by retraction (Summit, 1983), hence the necessity to videotape validation interviews. In a proportion of all child abuse cases, the non-abusing parent also denies the occurrence of the abuse.

Once the child is protected by a statutory order and a three column formulation has been constructed which offers an account of the pattern of interaction within which the abuse occurred, then a treatment contract may be offered. This may involve treatment approaches other than conjoint family meetings. With intrafamilial sexual abuse, one particularly effective programme has been developed by Hank Giaretto (1982) in Santa Clara, USA. The programme uses joint mother- daughter meetings to help mothers develop relationships with their abused children. Marital meetings are used to help the couple work through the conflict surrounding the abuse and establish an effective co-parenting relationship. Concurrently, fathers participate in highly confrontative group therapy with other sexual offenders to help them fully accept responsibility for their abuse of their daughters. Daughters participate in group assertiveness training and mothers participate in group therapy to help them work thorough their mixed feelings surrounding the abuse. Intermittent conjoint family meetings are also held. Families are only admitted to the programme if the father signs a confession admitting to the abuse, and non-compliance leads to immediate incarceration of the father. The programme is almost 100% successful.

With physical abuse, successful programmes use therapeutic contracts and focus on specific tasks such as helping parents develop the behaviour control and anger management skills necessary to break the escalating cycles of interaction around the presenting problem (Dale et al, 1986; Nicol et al, 1988). A variety of contextual factors, including social isolation, lack of social support, parental criminality, parental psychological adjustment difficulties, marital conflict and poverty have all been associated with physical child abuse. Successful programmes also address these issues on a per-case basis (Cicchetti and Carlson, 1989). However, there is also a wider political agenda here that needs to be addressed outside of the therapeutic arena.

With emotionally abused neglected children who show non-organic failure to thrive, a number of highly focused feeding based intervention programmes have been developed which are particularly effective (Hanks et al, 1988; Iwaniec et al, 1985).

MARITAL VIOLENCE

It was mentioned in Chapter 16, that when working with families referred for child-focused problems, often marital violence emerges as a central concern. Marital violence poses similar ethical dilemmas to those entailed by child abuse. In cases of marital violence, there is a conflict between the value of not condoning violence on the one hand and maintaining therapeutic neutrality on the other. If the therapist defines the violence in interactional terms there is a danger that this will amount to colluding with the aggressor, condoning the violence and partially blaming the victim. If the therapist blames the aggressor for the violent act, then this violates the principle of neutrality.

As with child abuse, denial is a feature of marital violence, often with both partners denying the occurrence of brutality. Individual therapy and marital work are usually deferred until child-focused problems have been dealt with in Positive Practice. However, marital violence is an exception to this rule.

When marital violence is seriously suspected, consultation cannot proceed without the parents agreeing to address the violence first. Willbach (1989) argues that family therapy should be abandoned unless the violent partner, usually the man, contracts for nonviolence. This intervention puts the responsibility for continuing treatment, not on the battered wife, but on the violent man. Bograd (1992) cautions that voluntary programmes for violent couples have poor success rates (about 30%), whereas those that occur as an alternative to a custodial sentence (much like Giaretto's sexual abuse programme described above) have a far better outcome. Useful accounts of treatment approaches are given in Goldner et al, 1990 and Deschner, 1984.

SECRETS

When one member of the problem-system reveals a secret to a therapist and asks that confidentiality be maintained, the therapist faces a dilemma. If this confidentiality is respected, then neutrality may be violated, particularly if the content of the secret is relevant to the maintenance or resolution of the presenting problem. In cases of child abuse, violence or self- harm, maintaining confidentiality about a secret may violate a commitment to minimizing harm and maximizing well-being. On the other hand if the therapist maintains neutrality by telling other family members about the secret, then the promise of confidentiality is broken. Before looking at the management of such situations let us first consider a useful typology of secrets.

Karpel (1980) distinguishes between individual secrets held by one person only; those shared by some, but not all family members; and family secrets which are known by all family members but are concealed from the community. A distinction may also be drawn between productive and destructive secrets. Individual secrets, in the form of a private daily journal or diary, may be productive insofar as they enrich the writer's sense of personal identity and autonomy. Shared secrets may be used to maintain boundaries between family subsystems. For example, many couples do not discuss the intimate details of their sexual relationship with their children. Here, shared secrets are productive by creating an integenerational boundary. Family secrets, such as preparing a surprise party for close friends, can generate joy and wonder.

Secrets are destructive where the withholding of information leads to a sense of guilt concerning the deception and this compromises the quality of important family relationships. With children and families, the most common example of this type of individual destructive secret is where a child has stolen something of particular value and concealed the theft. Less common, fortunately, is where the child has had ideas about self-injury which he or she has concealed. (Suicide and self-harm have already been discussed in Chapter 14.) Secrets are also destructive where the act of deception subjugates one or more members of the family, as in the case of intrafamilial sexual abuse. Such abuse is a typical example of a shared destructive secret. Some shared secrets, such as those related to adoptive children's parentage or a child's illegitimacy may be maintained by parents with the best of intentions but have a destructive impact on parent-child relationships when the child suspects deception. Destructive family secrets, such as those concerning family violence, often maintain problems by cutting the family off from people or agencies in the community that may be able to help the family.

When the therapist is offered a secret in confidence by a family member, in Positive Practice, the secret and the confidence are accepted and respected as a confused plea for help (Carpenter and Treacher, 1989, Chapter 5), not as attempts at therapeutic sabotage (Selvini-Palazzoli and Prata, 1982). The relevance of the secret to the maintenance and resolution of the presenting problems must then be established. Irrelevant secrets may be let lie. For example, the brother of a boy referred with learning difficulties mentioned to me, in confidence, in the waiting room that both boys had cheated in a school examination three years previously. This was acknowledged but not mentioned in later interviews because it was irrelevant to arranging for the family and school to manage the boy's learning difficulty more effectively. If the secret is relevant to the maintenance or resolution of the presenting problem, the implications for all family members of revealing or concealing it may be explored with the person who has revealed the secret. The father of a fourteen year old boy, Seamus, who was referred for stealing at school phoned me after the intake interview and said that his son was adopted, but that this had been kept a secret from him so that he would not feel like the black sheep of the family. There were two older non-adoptive sisters. I subsequently met with both parents to discuss this issue. Here are some of the questions that were used to explore the implications of concealing or revealing the secret.

- *Suppose you told Seamus, straight out, that you desperately wanted another child but couldn't have one so you adopted him, what do you guess would go through his mind?*
- *How do you think would go through his sister's minds?*
- *What is the worst thing that could happen if you told Seamus that he was adopted?*
- *In what way would your relationship with him change if you told him about this?*
- *In what way would the relationship between him and his sisters/aunts/granny/ grandad change if you told him about the adoption?*
- *For yourself, when you phoned me, how were you connecting Seamus' stealing and the fact that he was adopted?*

The main concern for the parents was that the process of adoption had disrupted Seamus' psychological development and that this was now finding expression through his stealing. They also moved from a position where they suspected that he would feel like an unwanted outsider if he knew about his adoption to a recognition that he might feel particularly valued, since his mother could not have further biological children. In a later highly emotional session the parents told Seamus about his adoption. This was a turning point in the therapy. From there on, the relationship, particularly between Seamus and his father improved markedly.

Where secrets concern violence or child abuse, the guidelines outlined in previous sections of this chapter may be followed. Secrets concerning self-harm may be managed in the way outlined in Chapter 14.

PARADOX AND DECEPTION

In cases that become stuck and in which defiance based paradoxical interventions may prove useful, a conflict may occur between the obligation to be honest with clients and the obligation to provide effective therapy (paradoxical tasks have been described in Chapter 9). If a defiance based paradoxical intervention is used and as a result the presenting problems are resolved, then the obligation to provide effective therapy has been met but the obligation to be honest has been violated. If the therapist honours a commitment to honesty, then the commitment to provide effective treatment may not be upheld.

Haley (1976) argued strongly that the therapist's ethical obligation to help clients resolve their problems as rapidly and efficiently as possible should be given priority over honesty. One difficulty with Haley's position is that, despite the impressive anecdotal reports, empirical evidence for the efficacy of paradoxical tasks is mixed (Shoham-Salomon and Rosenthal, 1987).

Wendorf and Wendorf (1985) argue that stating therapeutic dilemmas or using split messages from team members are more honest interventions that defiance based paradoxical tasks and yet serve a similar function. They capitalize upon clients' ambivalence about change. My own view is that the use of deception requires strong ethical justification in a particular case and greater empirical support more generally.

COMMENTS ON ETHICS AND POWER

Violence, secrets, deception and many other issues that raise ethical dilemmas are connected to the central concept of power. Within the field of family therapy there has been an ongoing debate about power, influence and responsibility since the 1950s when Gregory Bateson and Jay Haley first had a difference of opinion about this during the double bind project (Carr, 1991b; Jones, 1993, Chapter 7). Haley (1967; 1976a;b) argued that power is a central organizing construct in human interaction. In families and organizations people organize themselves into hierarchies. Many behavioural problems occur, according to Haley, when covert coalitions emerge which undermine overt hierarchies. For example, in many families referred for treatment a covert mother-child coalition may undermine the overt hierarchy which is deemed to exist between the parents at one level and the child at another. He also argued that therapy, while overtly a cooperative venture is covertly a power struggle. Because of this, he believed that the use of deception and paradox were ethically justified in helping clients resolve problems.

Bateson (1973) in contrast, argued that all people are involved in patterns of interaction characterized by mutual influence. Attempts to control the behaviour of others unilaterally may have devastating and unexpected consequences. Therefore, Bateson argued, the idea of power is not a useful construct for either explaining human interaction or for planning intervention. Rather, we should examine the characteristics of relationships by describing them as symmetrical, complimentary, or in some other relational way and construe therapy as a cooperative venture.

Within the family therapy field today, Selvini-Palazzoli (1986) in her dirty games project , feminists (e.g. McKinnon and Miller, 1987), and those concerned with social inequality and child abuse adopt a position reminiscent of Haley's. Cecchin's emphasis of cooperative co-construction in therapy (1987,1993) and Maturana and Varela's (1988) view on the impossibility of instructional interaction reflect Bateson's position.

Within Positive Practice, Bateson's notion of mutual influence is a central organizing idea. However, it is also recognized that mutuality of influence does not entail equality of influence. If a father, in exasperation, throws a screaming infant at the wall and the infant breaks his leg, the infant's crying has influenced the father and the father's frustration has influenced the child. Thus, there has been mutuality of influence. However, the impact of the child's influence on the father (making him frustrated) is not equal to the impact of the father's influence on the child (breaking a leg).

Haley's distinction between the overt and covert coalitions and agendas is particularly useful in the analysis of power relationships in families and resistance in therapy.

We have already referred to the pathological triangle in Chapter 3. More recently, Foucault's (1980) ideas of dominant and subjugated narratives have been imported into family therapy (White, 1993; Jones, 1993, Chapter 7). The idea that certain narratives become hierarchically superior to others which are suppressed and marginalized fits with Haley's analysis of power and is a useful idea when analysing the power structure of problem systems.

SUMMARY

An ethical dilemma is a situation where there is a conflict between two obligations, values or principles. In working with children and their families a number of situations commonly pose ethical dilemmas for clinicians. These include cases where child abuse and marital violence are suspected or have occurred. Cases where secrets are divulged to the therapist or where it appears that paradoxical interventions may be particularly helpful to the family also pose ethical dilemmas. Many of our ethical judgements are made intuitively without extensive conscious critical evaluation. An important factor contributing to the development of ethical intuition is the conscious critical evaluation and resolution of ethical dilemmas that have not been previously encountered by the clinician. Factors that inform critical evaluative ethical decision making include the practitioner's clinical model, their professional codes of ethics, the sociolegal context in which they work, their personal ethical principles and ethical theory. In Positive Practice, clinicians may look to each of these sources for guidance when faced with an ethical dilemma.

Exercise 17.1.

Work in pairs.

Begin by reading the following three situations.

1.   You discover facial bruising and a cigarette burn on Dawn Rooney (described in Exercise 2.1) during the third session with the family. Dawn attributes the bruise to a fall and you suspect child abuse.

2.   In an individual consultation Timmy Whitefriar (described in Exercise 4.1.) tells you that his parents are regularly violent to each other and asks you to keep this a secret.

3.   While working with the White family (mentioned in Exercise 13.2) you suspect that Barbara is being sexually abused by her father. The teachers say that she has hinted at this at school.

For each of the situations set out the ethical dilemma you face.

Outline the two main courses of action open to you.

Write down what your clinical model, professional codes of ethics, sociolegal context, personal ethical principles and ethical theory have to say about each of the alternative courses of action that are open to you.

Finally make an ethical decision.

Discuss the differences between the decisions reached by different group members.

18

Service Development and Professional Development

The process of checking that the type of consultation service that is offered in practice, matches the level and quality of the service that was intended is often referred to as clinical audit. It is useful to conduct this at both an individual case level and also at a global service level. At an individual case level, clinical audit answers the questions like:

- *In this case, how did the consultation process help the clients achieve their goals?*
- *If goals were not achieved, what went wrong?*
- *If the goals were achieved, how might the approach taken to consultation in this case be applied to other similar cases?*

Table 16.1 in Chapter 16, where the entire consultation process with the Barrows is summarized succinctly, is a typical example of an audit summary for an individual case. Considering this summary in the light of the three column formulation set out in Figure 7.1 and of the original contract would be a useful way to audit this case. This could be done by an individual therapist, a clinical team, or a group of professional peers. Professional peer review meetings are particularly valuable, because they provide a forum within which colleagues can receive feedback on their clinical work from other therapists.

At a more global level, clinical audit aims to determine if the overall service is meeting the targets it was designed to meet and to suggest avenues for service development. Most centres have an implicit or explicit aim to provide a particular sort of service for a particular population. Most services also have views on who should refer cases, what level of staff input should occur per case and what level of therapeutic success, client satisfaction and referrer satisfaction are acceptable. To check if these implicit or explicit targets or criteria are being reached it is useful to design an audit system to answer the following sorts of questions.

- *Who refers clients for consultation?*
- *With what type of problems do they want help?*
- *What are the socio-demographic characteristics of the clients?*
- *How many cases are seen for consultation per year?*
- *How many achieve their goals?*
- *How many dropout before the end of the consultation contract?*
- *How many hours of staff input occur per case?*
- *Who is usually the main customer for consultation?*
- *How satisfied are clients and referrers with the service offered?*
- *What factors are related to staff input and case outcome?*
- *How may the service be improved?*
- *How may the service be developed to meet the needs of subgroups of clients or referrers?*

In Figures 18.1, 18.2 and 18.3, audit forms for completion by clinicians, clients and referrers are presented. This set of forms constitutes an audit system for use in a Child and Family Centre. Let us examine them one by one. The form in Figure 18.1 is completed by the therapist. It collects information on the source of the referral (item 2) and also on the main customer as identified by the therapist (item 8). Both are included since information about who refers the case and who wants help are both useful for planning how clients may access the service. The items that collect information on case-type; the age and sex of the identified problem child; the family type and the family's socio-economic status are useful since they offer a profile of the client group served and so may have implications for the way in which the service is developed to target particular subgroups in the future. Some of these client-profile items may also be related to outcome or to the number of hours of staff input per case. This type of information is useful when planning the type of case-mix a clinic as a whole should try to service, and also when planning individual clinicians' workloads. For example, in an audit myself and my colleagues in Norfolk conducted, about a third of our cases were classified as complex and multiproblem (Carr et al, 1994).

These consumed a substantial portion of the staff's time. However, it was part of the Centre's policy to give priority to such cases, since local treatment alternatives were unavailable for these cases, whereas some alternatives were available for cases with focal problems. A particularly interesting finding from our audit was that classifying cases as having focal or multiple problems was more useful, from the point of view of service planning, than using other descriptors such as diagnosis.

Items 9 and 10 of the Clinic Audit Form collect data on whether assessment and therapy phases of the consultation process were completed and the degree to which goals were attained. Thus, they furnish information on outcome from the therapist's perspective. Information on improvement in the presenting problem from the client's and referrer's perspective are furnished by the first item both on the Client Audit Form and on the Referrer's Audit Form.

Scores on items 2, 3 and 4 of the Client Audit Form may be summed to produce an index of the client's satisfaction with the service offered. The three items have been adapted from Larsen's (1979) Client Satisfaction Scale. (Larsen's original three items, which were written for individuals, emerged as the briefest reliable and valid scale from a psychometric analysis of eighty-one items.) Scores on items 2, 3 and 4 of the Referrer Audit Form may be summed to give an index of referrer satisfaction.

INFORMATION	VARIABLE		COMPUTER CODE
Names_____ _____ Address_____ _____ Phone_____	CASE IDENTIFICATION DETAILS AND NUMBER		1. Case Identity
Referrer_____ Address_____ _____ _____ _____ Phone_____	REFERRAL SOURCE Self GP School Hospital Social services Other	1 2 3 4 5 6	2. Referrer
Main problem and Involved agencies _____	CASE TYPE Focal problem Complex multiproblem	1 2	3. Case type
Family composition	FAMILY TYPE Unmarried couple First marriage Unmarried single parent Separated single parent Reconstituted family	1 2 3 4 5	4. Family type
Identified problem person Name_____ Age_____ Sex_____	AGE in years		5. Age
	SEX Male Female	0	6. Sex
Parent's occupations Father's_____ _____ Mother's_____ _____	SOCIO-ECONOMIC STATUS Higher prof/Manager Lower prof/Manager Non manual (other) Skilled manual Semiskilled Unskilled Unemployed	1 2 3 4 5 6 7	7. SES
Main customer _____ _____ _____ _____ _____	CUSTOMER Child Parents GP School Hospital Social services Other	1 2 3 4 5 6 7	8. Customer
Assessment completed and formulation agreed	ASSESSMENT Yes No (dropped out)	1 0	9. Assessment
Therapy contract goals _____ _____ _____ _____ _____	THERAPY Therapy not offered (assessment only) Dropout Minimal goal attainment Partial goal attainment Complete goal attainment	0 1 2 3 4	10. Therapy
Number of hours input including family sessions, network consultation, telephone contact etc.	STAFF INPUT IN HOURS		11. Hours

Figure 18.1. Child and family clinic audit form

You recently attended our service with your family. We are writing to ask for your help. We want to improve the service we offer

to families. So we would value your opinion and that of another member of your family on the service you received. Please fill

out this form and ask one other family member to complete the other enclosed form. Then return them to us in the enclosed

stamped addressed envelope. Thank you.

Please **circle your answer** to each of the following questions

1. Have the problems that led to you coming to our service improved?	No they are worse 1	No they are the same 2	Yes there is some improvement 3	Yes there is a lot of Improvement 4
2. To what extent has our service met your family's needs?	None of our needs have been met 1	Only a few of our needs have been met 2	Most of our needs have been met 3	Almost all of our needs have been met 4
3. In an overall general sense, how satisfied are you with the service you received?	Quite dissatisfied 1	Mildly satisfied 2	Mostly satisfied 3	Very satisfied 4
4. If your family wanted help again, would you come back to our service?	No. definitely not. 1	No I don't think so 2	Yes I think so 3	Yes definitely 4
5. When your family was coming to the clinic, did you want to come?	No. definitely not. 1	No not really 2	Yes a little 3	Yes definitely 4
6. What is your role in the family?	Mother	Father	Child	Other

What was most helpful about coming to the Child and Family Clinic?

What was least helpful about coming to the Child and Family Clinic?

Figure 18.2.   Child and family service client audit form

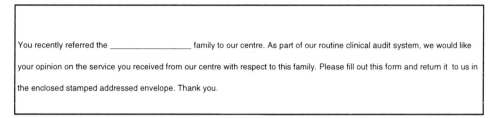

You recently referred the _____ family to our centre. As part of our routine clinical audit system, we would like your opinion on the service you received from our centre with respect to this family. Please fill out this form and return it to us in the enclosed stamped addressed envelope. Thank you.

Please **circle your answer** to each of the following questions

1 Have the problems that led to the referral of this family improved?	No they are worse 1	No they are the same 2	Yes there is some improvement 3	Yes There is a lot of improvement 4
2 To what extent has our service met the family's needs?	None of our needs have been met 1	Only a few of our needs have been met 2	Most of our needs have been met 3	Almost all of our needs have been met 4
3 In an overall general sense, how satisfied are you with the service we provided for the family and yourself as the referrer?	Quite dissatisfied 1	Mildly satisfied 2	Mostly satisfied 3	Very satisfied 4
4 If you wanted to refer this or similar families for help in the future would you refer to our service?	No definitely not 1	No I don't think so 2	Yes I think so 3	Yes definitely 4
5 Have you had to provide the family with less of **YOUR TIME**, since referring the case to our centre?	No definitely not 1	No I don't think so 2	Yes I think so 3	Yes definitely 4
6 Has the **RISK** of abuse or self-injury been reduced since the referral (if it is a self-harm or child protection case)?	Not applicable 0	No definitely not 1	possibly 2	Yes definitely 3
7 Has the **MANAGEMENT** of the case become **SIMPLER** since the referral (if this is a complex multiproblem case with many agencies involved)?	Not applicable 0	No definitely not 1	possibly 2	Yes definitely 3
8 Who was most concerned that the referral be made originally?	Myself 1	The family 2	The school 3	Social services 4

If you have comments on the **most and least helpful aspects of our service** please put them on the back of this form. Thank you.

Figure 18.3. Child and family service referrer audit form

Items 5 and 6 of the Client Audit Form give information on the degree to which the client was a customer for consultation and on their role in the family. Information on the referrer's perception of the main customer for consultation is obtained through item 8 of the Referrer's Audit Form.

The lessening of a referrer's perception of a case as extremely complex to manage or as posing a risk of child abuse or violence have been identified as important indices of the usefulness of systemic consultation to statutory social workers who refer cases for family consultation (Manor, 1991). For this reason, Items 6 and 7 have been included in the Referrer Audit Form. Item 5, which assesses the degree to which systemic consultation reduces the amount of time the referrer has to devote to the case, was identified by GPs as a valuable index of the usefulness of a consultation service for children and families (Carr, McDonnell and Owen, 1994).

On both the Client and Referrer Audit Forms an opportunity is given for the respondent to comment on the most and least helpful aspects of the service. This qualitative data may suggest particular ways in which aspects of the consultation process or service delivery system may be improved.

The three forms have been developed in the light of the available literature on audit in the child and family mental health field and of our own experience with audit in a busy child and family clinic (Berger et al, 1993; Carr, McDonnell and Owen, 1994). Of course, the forms will probably require some local modifications if you want to use them within your practice. However, if you do modify them, it is worth keeping in mind the criteria that were used during their development. First, the forms collect essential information only. Many available audit systems are wonderfully comprehensive (e.g. Berger et al, 1993). However, our experience is that, after an initial rush of enthusiasm, staff forget to fill out large comprehensive audit forms and clients do not return them. Second, the forms are designed so that the information from them may easily be entered into a computer database. The information on the Clinic Audit Form may be converted to eleven computer code numbers in the right hand column. Information from the Client Audit Forms may be computer coded as six numbers: one for each item. Information from the Referrer Audit Form may be entered into a computer database as eight number codes. The third feature of the system is that it is compact. Each form is only a single side of a single page. The fourth, important characteristic of the system is that it is as simple and unambiguous as possible. The final attribute of the system deserving mention is its user-friendliness for staff, referrers and clients.

All three audit forms may be used with every case. However, this may be time consuming and expensive. A good compromise is to complete a clinic audit form on every case and to invite a subsample of referrers and clients to complete audit forms.

Information from this audit system if analysed using simple database software may be fruitfully used to produce periodic audit reports. The open ended comments from clients and referrers may be used to compliment the quantitative information produced by the database analyses. For example, you may find that 80% of clients and 70% of referrers were satisfied with the service. A common remark from clients may have been that the thing they most liked about the service was the fact that everybody in the family was given a fair hearing. On the other hand referrers may have found the short waiting list the most helpful aspect of the service. This mixing of quantitative and qualitative data can offer a rounded picture of the degree to which a service meets the targets it set out to achieve and offer useful suggestions on avenues for service development.

It has already been mentioned that audit allows clinicians to check if they are offering the type of service that they intend to offer, and that audit also points to ways in which the service may be developed and practice enhanced. This recursive relationship between practice and audit is diagrammed in Figure 18.4. Audit reports are also useful documents to use in support of applications for resources to management, funding agencies and service purchasers. Unfortunately, family therapy as a movement has been quick to make unsubstantiated claims for its effectiveness as a panacea for all ills, and slow to establish a body of empirical research data to back these claims or to equip

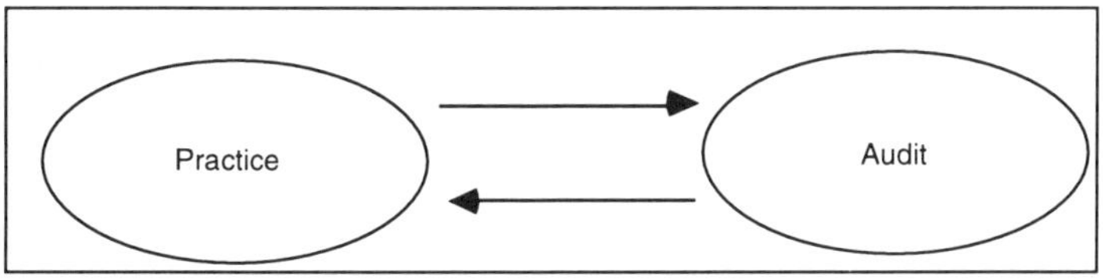

Figure 18.4.   The relationship between audit and practice

practitioners with audit skills through which to demonstrate the effectiveness of their particular service (Carr, 1991a). The simple audit system presented in this chapter offers clinicians a way out of this dilemma.

AN EXAMPLE OF A CLINICAL AUDIT AND ITS IMPACT

This audit (Carr, McDonnell and Owen, 1994) of practice at a child and family centre included a sixteen month case note review covering 319 cases, a postal survey of 45 families and an interview survey of 10 GPs who typically referred cases to the centre. The audit furnished information from three different perspectives on the referral process, the consultation process, and the outcome for clients attending the centre. The referral rate was about one new case per day, and peak referral times were the beginning of the autumn and winter school terms. Almost half the referrals came from GPs and the remainder were largely from Paediatrics, Education and Social Services. Most clients were seen within two months. Half of the families referred had serious psychosocial difficulties, including multiple problem members, multiproblem children, multi-agency involvement, psychoeducational difficulties, child protection problems or child placement difficulties. The majority of cases received six hours of consultation. Families where child abuse had occurred or families containing a multiproblem adolescent received a more intensive service. Between one half and three quarters of cases had positive outcomes as rated by staff and parents. The service was viewed by GPs to be highly satisfactory. On the negative side, many parents felt ill-prepared for the consultation process, and most children did not enjoy the experience. This audit data evoked a number of responses.

First, we were surprised that half of the families we saw presented with multiple problems and represented a client group with serious and extensive therapeutic needs. We had not suspected that the proportion was so large. Second, we were pleased to note that, despite the large proportion of our cases that fell into the multiproblem category, our successful outcome rate was in keeping with the results of controlled treatment outcome studies (e.g. Carr, 1991a). This information, along with the statistics on referral rate of one new family per day or over 1,000 new people per year was useful in making a case to management about increasing staffing levels. Third, we were disap-pointed that many of the families that were referred to us felt ill-prepared for the consultation process. We took steps to rectify this situation by writing an extensive services prospectus and making this available to referring agents. Fourth, we were also disappointed to learn that children found the consultation process unpleasant. The approach to individual consultations described in Chapter 14 was more explicitly formulated in response to the negative feedback concerning children's perception of the consultation process.

PROFESSIONAL AND PERSONAL DEVELOPMENT

Clinical audit provides signposts which establish a direction for service development and the enhancement of practice. However, continuing professional development (CPD) is vital if clinicians are to empower themselves to follow the leads suggested by audit.

A CPD PROGRAMME SHOULD

1.   Empower you to translate conceptual, perceptual and practical skills into Positive Practice
2.   Provide emotional support
3.   Challenge you to explore emotional blind-spots
4.   Help you to manage competing demands
5.   Help you to plan your career

Figure 18.5.   Characteristics of a good continuing professional development programme

A good CPD programme should provide you with the ingredients listed in Figure 18.5. Each of these will be discussed in some detail below. However, let me first clarify that a CPD programme is a planned series of activities which aim to enhance professional development in an ongoing way. Such a programme may include, for example, membership of a peer supervision group; regular reading of professional journals and books; attendance at conferences, workshops or training courses; and personal psychotherapy. When you plan your own CPD programme, it is important that you achieve a good balance of all of the ingredients listed in Figure 18.5. Let us now turn to the first of these.

A CPD programme should provide you with technical skills training. That is, it should help you to develop and renew your conceptual, perceptual and practical therapeutic skills and translate these into Positive Practice (Tomm, 1979). Conceptual skills are those which we use to organize information about our work. For example, being able to use the three column formulation model to integrate information about a case is a conceptual skill. The ability to attend selectively to particular features of a case, such as patterns of interaction around a symptom, is a good example of a perceptual skill. Practical skills are those which we use when we conduct interviews or convene meetings.

Second, a CPD programme should provide you with the emotional support necessary to continue to work closely with a demanding caseload without burning out. Burnout is a very common phenomenon among health care professionals (Maslach and Jackson, 1982). Maslach identifies three main components to the burnout syndrome: emotional exhaustion, a belief that one is professionally or clinically impotent, and a tendency to avoid emotional or physical proximity to clients. Let us look at each of these components. Emotional exhaustion is the feeling of being completely drained and unable to engage with clients at an emotional level to offer help with problems of living. The second component of burnout is the belief that you are unable to help clients achieve their goals and solve the problems with which they require help. This may be due to an awareness that you cannot join with clients because of emotional exhaustion. The third component of burnout is avoidance of emotional or physical contact with clients. This often involves treating clients as if they were objects rather than people and so has been termed depersonalization.

Burnout is related to the therapist's belief system, skill level and behavioural style, and also to the culture and characteristics of the organization in which the therapist works (Fruggeri, and McNamee, 1991). Many people are attracted into the helping professions because they have a strong need to help others. This may be because they believe that those they help will repay them with gratitude and that this gratitude will meet unresolved dependency needs. This type of belief system can lead to burnout where therapists lack of skill, large and difficult case loads and organizational factors, such as lack of supervision and support, prevent therapists from helping clients effectively. This situation cuts therapists off from the gratitude they require to satisfy unmet dependency needs. Even if therapists are not *gratitude junkies*, organizational cultures that do not have a policy for dealing with the engagement difficulties listed in Chapter 2, that value therapists servicing large caseloads in relative isolation and that overemphasize the therapist's responsibility in promoting problem resolution, can lead to burnout.

Burnout usually spills over into homelife and has a negative impact on family and marital relationships. Therapists who are emotionally exhausted and who believe that they have failed in their professional lives may have little left to contribute to family life other than irritability or withdrawal. Alcohol, and drug usage provide a haven where burntout therapists can escape from the pain of the condition. Fortunately, burnout need not be a permanent state. Those of us who have been through it, know that it is temporary and within the context of a good CPD programme, the experience of burnout can teach us a lot about our strengths as well as our vulnerabilities.

A third feature of a good CPD programme is that it provides you with the challenge to explore emotional blind-spots and countertransference reactions evoked by working in difficult therapeutic systems. All of us have particular situations, emotions and patterns of interaction that we automatically avoid or approach. Sometimes these unconscious habits, which we usually learn in our early life, prevent us from helping clients. If we unconsciously avoid issues related to loss, conflict, confusion, sexuality, anger, sadness, or anxiety we may be compromised in our capacity to offer flexible consultation when these issues emerge. Similarly, if we are drawn to establish complimentary relationships with needy clients or symmetrical relationships with angry clients then these habits will constrain our flexibility in finding solutions to presenting problems. The exploration of these types of approach-avoidance habits is an important part of a useful CPD programme.

A fourth characteristic of a good CPD programme is that it must provide a way for you to consider how best to situate yourself among the competing demands of work and home life; colleagues, managers and policy makers; clients, referrers and team members; line staff and trainees. This complex personal network may be visualized as Figure 18.6. In Chapter 2, engagement mistakes that can occur when therapists are over-focused on the family as the unit of treatment and fail to take account of the wider professional network were discussed. This is just one example of a set of problems that may arise from the exclusive focus on one aspect of your own network to the exclusion of others. Implicit in the earlier discussion of burnout, was the idea that therapists who devote

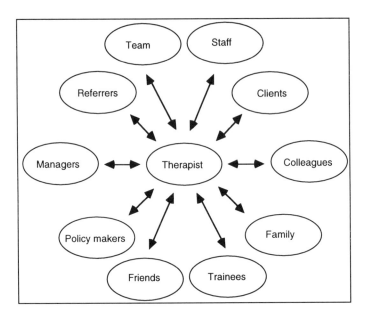

Figure 18.6.   The therapist's network

themselves almost exclusively to case management, without regard to their organizational context and family life, run the risk of exacerbating their sense of exhaustion. When work based difficulties arise that involve more than one case, a useful CPD programme provides a context within which you can map out the pattern of interaction around the problem and the related beliefs of all involved with due regard to members of all the subsystems charted in Figure 18.6.

Finally, a CPD programme must provide a periodic forum within which to keep track of your overall career plan. Professionals who practice systemic consultation may have many potential career avenues open in the public and private sectors. Career opportunities are available in medical, social, educational, religious, law enforcement, rehabilitation and business contexts. Systemic consultation offers opportunities in clinical practice, training and supervision, and in research and policy development. A CPD programme should offer you occasional opportunities to take stock of what you have done and to consider future options.

POSITIVE PRACTICE: A FINAL WORD

Positive Practice is an approach to systemic consultation and family therapy where new developments in theory, research and training are continually translated into practical procedures. This book is therefore no more than a signpost pointing to a way you may choose to organize your own integrative approach to systemic consultation.

Good luck.

Exercise 18.1.

Work in pairs.

Plan an audit system for your practice.

Discuss the feasibility of implementing this with the group.

Exercise 18.2.

Work in pairs (interviewer/interviewee).

Conduct an interview in which a personal CPD plan is constructed for the interviewee.

This CPD plan must meet the criteria set out in Figure 18.5.

Swap roles and repeat the exercise.

Discuss the obstacles to implementing these plans in a group and brainstorm ways around these blocks.

References

Abramson, L., Seligman, M. and Teasdale, J. (1978) Learned helplessness in humans: Critique and reformulation. *Journal of Abnormal Psychology*, 87, 49–74.

Ainsworth, M. , Blehar, M., Waters, E. and Wall, S. (1978) *Patterns of Attachment. A Psychological Study of Strange Situations.* Hillsdale, NJ: Lawrence Erlbaum.

American Psychiatric Association (1994) *DSM-IV* Washington, DC: APA.

Andersen, T. (1987) Reflecting teams: Dialogue and metalogue in clinical work. *Family Process*, 26, 415–428.

Anderson, C. and Stewart, S. (1983) *Mastering Resistance.* New York: Guilford.

Anderson, H., Goolishan, H. and Windermand, L. (1986) Problem determined systems: Toward transformation in family therapy. *Journal of Strategic and Systemic Therapies*, 5 (4), 1–14.

Bandura, A. (1981) Self-efficacy mechanisms in human agency. *American Psychologist*, 37, 122–147.

Barker, P. (1986) *Basic Family Therapy. 2nd edition.* Oxford: Blackwell.

Barker, P. (1988) *Basic Child Psychiatry. 5th edition.* Oxford: Blackwell.

Barton, C. and Alexander, J. (1981) Functional family therapy. In A. Gurman, and D. Kniskern (eds.) *Handbook of Family Therapy.* New York: Brunner/Mazel.

Bateson, G. (1973) *Steps to an Ecology of Mind.* St Albans: Paladin.

Beck, A. and Steer, R. (1991) *Beck Scale for Suicide Ideation.* New York: The Psychological Corporation.

Beck, A. and Weishaar, M. (1989) Cognitive therapy. In R. Corsini and D. Wedding (eds.) *Current Psychotherapies. 4th edition.* Ithaca, Ill. Peacock.

Bennun, I. (1989). Perceptions of the therapist in family therapy. *Journal of Family Therapy*, 11, 243–255.

Berger, M., Hill, P., Sein, E., Thompson, M. and Verduyn, C. (1993) *A Proposed Core Data Set for Child and Adolescent Psychology and Psychiatry Services.* London: Association for Child Psychology and Psychiatry.

Berman, A. and Jobes, D. (1993) *Adolescent suicide: Assessment and intervention.* Washington DC: APA.

Bograd, M. (1992) Values in conflict: Challenges to family therapists thinking. *Journal of Marital and Family Therapy*, 18, 245–256.

Breunlin, D. (1994) Developments in family therapy in the USA. Special edition of *Journal of Family Therapy*, 16, 1–142.

Byng-Hall, J. (1988) Scripts and legends in family therapy. *Family Process*, 27, 167–179.

Campbell, D., Draper, R. and Crutchley, E. (1991) The Milan Systemic Approach to Family Therapy. In A. Gurman, and D. Kniskern (eds.) *Handbook of Family Therapy. Volume 2*. New York: Brunner/Mazel.

Carl, D. and Jurkovic, G. (1983) Agency triangles: Problems in agency-family relationships. *Family Process*, 22, 441–451.

Carpenter, J. and Treacher, A. (1989). *Problems and Solutions in Marital and Family Therapy*. Oxford: Basil Blackwell.

Carr, A. (1986) Three techniques for the solo-family therapist. *Journal of Family Therapy*, 8, 373–382.

Carr, A. (1989) Countertransference reactions to families where child abuse has occurred. *Journal of Family Therapy*, 11, 87–97.

Carr, A. (1990a) Failure in family therapy: A catalogue of engagement mistakes. *Journal of Family Therapy*, 12, 371–386.

Carr, A. (1990b) A formulation model for use in family therapy. *The Australian and New Zealand Journal of Family Therapy*, 11, 85–92.

Carr, A. (1990c) Giving directives effectively: The implications of research on compliance with doctor's orders for family therapy. *Human Systems: Journal of Systemic Consultation and Management*, 1, 115–127.

Carr, A. (1990d) Compliance with medical advice. *British Journal of General Practice*, 40 (No. 338), 358-360.

Carr, A. (1990e) From Problem to Solution. Report on a workshop by Steve de Shazer and Insoo Kim Berg from the Milwalkee Brief Therapy Centre, USA. *Context*, Summer, No. 6, 12–15.

Carr, A. (1991a) Milan Systemic Family Therapy: A review of 10 empirical investigations. *Journal of Family Therapy*, 13, 237–264.

Carr, A. (1991b) Power and influence in systemic consultation. *Human Systems: Journal of Systemic Consultation and Management*, 2, 15–30.

Carr, A. (1993) Systemic consultation and goal setting. *Human Systems :The Journal of Systemic Consultation and Management*, 4, 49–59.

Carr, A. (1994a) Family Psychology. The emergence of a new field. *Thornfield Journal*, 17, 1–8.

Carr, A. (1994b) Involving children in family therapy and systemic consultation. *Journal of Family Psychotherapy*, 5, 41–59.

Carr, A. and Afnan, S. (1989) Concurrent individual and family therapy in a case of elective mutism. *Journal of Family Therapy*, 11, 29–44.

Carr, A., Gawlinski, G., MacDonnell, D., Irving, N., and Docking, S. (1989) Thurlow House Adolescent Assessment Programme. *Practice*, 2, 60–190.

Carr, A. MacDonnell, D., and Afnan, S. (1989) Anorexia nervosa: The treatment of a male case with combined behavioural and family therapy. *Journal of Family Therapy*, 11, 335–351.

Carr, A. McDonnell, D. and Owen, P. (1994) Audit and family systems consultation: Evaluation of practice at a child and family centre. *Journal of Family Therapy*, 16, 143–157.

Carter, E. and McGoldrick, M. (1989) *The Family Lifecycle: A framework for family therapy. 2nd edition* Boston: Allyn and Bacon.

Cecchin, G. (1987) Hypothesizing, circularity and neutrality revisited: An invitation to curiosity. *Family Process*, 26, 405–413.

Cecchin, G., Lane, G. and Wendle, R. (1993). From strategising to non-intervention: Toward irreverence in systemic practice. *Journal of marital and Family Therapy*, 2, 125–136.

Chess, S. and Thomas, A. (1984). *Origins and Evolution of Behaviour Disorder from Infancy to Early Adult Life*. New York: Brunner/Mazel

Cicchetti, D. and Carlson, V. (1989) *Child Maltreatment.* Cambridge: Cambridge University Press.

Clarke-Finnegan, M. and Fahy, T. (1983) *Suicide rates in Ireland. Psychological Medicine,* 13, 385–391.

Colapinto, J. (1991). Structural Family Therapy. In A. Gurman, and D. Kniskern (eds) *Handbook of Family Therapy. Volume 2.* New York: Brunner/Mazel.

Coleman, S. (1985) *Failures in Family Therapy.* New York: Guilford.

Colgan, I. (1991)*The Fifth Province Model: Father-Daughter Incest Disclosure and Systemic Consultation.* Unpublished PhD Thesis, University College Dublin, National University of Ireland.

Critchfield, T. (1989) Self-recording mutually exclusive multiple responses. *Behaviour Modification,* 13, 361–375.

Cronen, V. and Pearse, B. (1985) Toward an explanation of how the Milan Method works. An invitation to a systemic epistemology and the evolution of family systems. In D. Campbell and R. Draper (eds) *Applications of Systemic Family Therapy: The Milan Approach.* London: Grune Stratton.

Crowther, C., Dare, C. and Wilson, J. (1990) 'Why should I talk to you? You'll only tell the court!' On being an informer and a family therapist. *Journal of Family Therapy,* 12, 105–122.

Cummings, C., Gordon, J. and Marlatt, A. (1980) Relapse:prevention and prediction. In W. Miller (ed.) *The Addictive Behaviours.* Oxford: Pergamon.

Dale, P. (1986) *Dangerous Families: Assessment and Treatment of Child Abuse.* London: Tavistock.

DeKraai, M. and Sales, B. (1991) Legal issues in the conduct of child therapy. In T. Kratchowill and R. Morris (eds) *The Practice of Child Therapy.* New York: Pergammon.

Deschner, J. (1984) *The Hitting Habit: Anger Control for Battering Couples.* New York Free Press.

deShazer, S. (1985) *Keys to solutions in brief therapy.* New York: Norton.

deShazer, S. (1988) *Clues: Investigating Solutions in Brief Therapy.* New York: Norton.

Dimmock, B. and Dungworth, D. (1985) Beyond the Family. Using network meetings with statutory child care cases. *Journal of Family Therapy,* 7, 45–68.

Dusay, J. and Dusay, C. (1989). Transactional Analysis. In R. Corsini and D. Wedding (eds) *Current Psychotherapies. 4th edition.* Ithaca, Ill: Peacock.

Epstein, N., and Bishop, D. (1981) Problem centred systems therapy of the family. In A. Gurman, and D. Kniskern (eds) *Handbook of Family Therapy.* New York: Brunner/Mazel.

Falloon, I. (1991) Behavioural Family Therapy. In A. Gurman, and D. Kniskern (eds) *Handbook of Family Therapy. Volume 2.* New York: Brunner/Mazel.

Falloon, I. Laporta, M., Fadden, G. and Graham-Hole, V. (1993). *Managing Stress in Families.* London: Routledge.

Foucault, M. (1980) *Power/Knowledge: Selected interviews and other writings* (Edited by C. Gordon). New York: Harvester Wheatsheaf.

Frank, J. (1967) *Persuasion and Healing.* Baltimore: Johns Hopkins Press.

Friedman, E. (1991) Bowen theory and therapy. In A. Gurman, and D. Kniskern (eds) *Handbook of Family Therapy. Volume 2.* New York: Brunner/Mazel.

Fruggeri, L. and McNamee, S. (1991) Burnout as social process: A research study. In L. Fruggeri, U. Telfner, A. Castellucci, M. Maurizio, and M. Matteine (eds) *New Systemic Ideas From the Italian Mental Health Movement.* London: Karnac Books.

Fulero, S. (1988) *Tarasoff:* Ten years later. *Professional Psychology,* 19, 84-90.

Giaretto, H. (1882) A comprehensive child sexual abuse treatment programme. *Child Abuse and Neglect,* 6, 263–278.

Gilligan, R. (1991) *Irish Child Care Services: Policy, Practice, and Provision.* Dublin: IPA.

Gilligan, S. and Price, R. (1993) *Therapeutic Conversations.* New York: Norton.

Goldner, V., Penn., P., Sheinberg, M. and Walker, G. (1990) Love and violence: Gender paradoxes in volatile attachments. *Family Process,* 29, 343–364.

Guttman, H. (1991) Systems Theory, Cybernetics and Epistemology. In A. Gurman, and D. Kniskern (eds) *Handbook of Family Therapy. Volume 2.* New York: Brunner/Mazel.

Haley, J. (1967) Towards a theory of pathological Systems. In G. Zuk and I. Boszormenyi Nagi (eds) *Family Therapy and Disturbed Families.* Palo Alto, CA: Science and Behaviour.

Haley, J. (1973) *Uncommon Therapy.* New York: Norton.

Haley, J. (1976a) *Problem solving therapy.* New York: Harper and Row.

Haley, J. (1976b). Development of a theory: A history of a research project. In C. Sluzki and D. Ransom (eds) *Double Bind: Foundation of the Communicational Approach to the Family.* New York: Grune and Stratton.

Haley, J. (1980) *Leaving Home.* New York: McGraw Hill.

Hanks, H., Hobbs, C., Seymour, D. and Stratton, P. (1988) Infants who fail to thrive: An intervention for poor feeding practices. *Journal of Reproductive and Infant Psychology,* 6, 101–111.

Hawton, K. (1992) Attempted suicide in children and adolescents. *Journal of Child Psychology and Psychiatry,* 23, 497–503.

Hawton, K. and Catalan, J. (1982) *Attempted Suicide: A Practical Guide to its Nature and Management.* Oxford: Oxford University Press.

Heath, A. (1985) Ending family therapy sessions: Some new directions. *Family Therapy Collections,* 14, 33–40.

Hederman, M. and Kearney, R. (1982)*The Crane Bag. Book of Irish Studies.* Dublin: Blackwater Press.

Herbert, M. (1987) *Behaviour Treatment of Children with Problems. 2nd edition.* London: Academic Press.

Herbert, M., (1991) *Clinical Child Psychology.* Chichester: Wiley.

Hersov, L. (1985) School refusal. In M. Rutter and L. Hersov (eds) *Child and Adolescent Psychiatry. Modern Approaches. 2nd edition.* Oxford: Blackwell.

Hoffman, L. (1990) From system to discourse. *Human Systems: The Journal of Systemic Consultation and Management,* 1, 4–8.

Hoffman, S. and Gafni, S. (1985) Active interactional co-therapy. *International Journal of Family Therapy,* 6, 53–58.

Hogbin, B. and Fallowfield, L. (1989) Getting it taped: The 'bad news' consultation with cancer patients. *British Journal of Hospital Medicine,* 41, 330–333.

Howe, D. (1989) *Consumer's Views of Family Therapy.* Aldershot, Hants: Gower.

Imber-Black, E. (1991) A family-larger-system-perspective. In A. Gurman, and D. Kniskern (eds) *Handbook of Family Therapy .Volume 2.* New York: Brunner/Mazel.

Ioannou, C. (1991) Acute pain in children. In M. Herbert (ed.) *Clinical Child Psychology.* Chichester: Wiley.

Iwaniec, D., Herbert, M. and McNeish, S. (1985) Social work with failure to thrive children and their families. *British Journal of Social Work,* 15, 375 389.

Jenkins, H. (1989) Precipitating crises in families: Patterns which connect. *Journal of Family Therapy,* 11, 99–109.

Jones, D. and McQuiston, M. (1983) *Interviewing the Sexually Abused Child.* London: Gaskell.

Jones, E. (1993) *Family Systems Therapy.* Chichester: Wiley.

Joyce, J. (1922)*Ulysses.* Middlesex: Penguin.

Karpel, M. (1980) Family Secrets: 1. Conceptual and ethical issues in the relational context. 11. Ethical and practical considerations in therapeutic management. *Family Process,* 19, 295–306.

Karpman, S. (1968) Fairy tales and script drama analysis. *Transactional Analysis Bulletin,* 7 (26), 39–44.

Kazdin, A. (1991) Aggressive behaviour and conduct disorder. In T. Kratchowill and R. Morris (eds) *The Practice of Child Therapy.* New York: Pergammon.

Kelly, G. (1955) *The Psychology of Personal Constructs. Volumes 1 and 2.* New York: Norton.

Kenny, V. (ed.) (1988) Radical Constructivism, Autopoesis and Psychotherapy. Special edition of *Irish Journal of Psychology*, 9 (1).

Korner, S. and Brown, G. (1990) Exclusion of children from family psychotherapy: Family therapists beliefs and practices. *Journal of Family Psychology*, 3, 420–430.

Kratchowill, T and Morris, R. (1991) *The Practice of Child Therapy.* New York: Pergammon.

L'Abate, L. and Jurkovic, G. (1987) Family systems theory as a cult: Boom or Bankruptcy. In L. L'Abate (ed.) *Family Psychology II. Theory, Therapy, Enrichment and Training.* Lanham: University Press of America.

Lang, P., Little, M. and Cronen, V. (1990) The systemic professional: Domains of action and the question of neutrality. *Human Systems: The Journal of Systemic Consultation and Management*, 1, 39–55.

Lankton, S., Lankton, C. and Matthews, W. (1991) Ericksonian family therapy. In A. Gurman, and D. Kniskern (eds) *Handbook of Family Therapy. Volume 2.* New York: Brunner/Mazel.

Larsen, D., Attkisson, C., Hargreaves, W. and Nguyen, T. (1979) Assessment of client/patient satisfaction: Development of a general scale. *Evaluation and Programme Planning*, 2, 197–207.

Lask, B. and Matthew, D. (1979) Childhood asthma: A controlled trial of family psychotherapy. *Archives of Disease in Childhood*, 54, 116–119.

Levy, S. and Heiden, L. (1991) Depression, distress and immunity: Risk factors for infectious disease. *Stress Medicine*, 7, 45–51.

Macrae, A. (1978) Forensic psychiatry. In A. Forrest, J. Affleck and A. Zealley (eds) *Companion to Psychiatric Studies.* Edinburgh: Churchill Livingstone.

Madanes, C. (1991) Strategic Family Therapy. In A. Gurman, and D. Kniskern (eds) *Handbook of Family Therapy. Volume 2.* New York: Brunner/Mazel.

Malan, D. (1979) *Individual Psychotherapy and the Science of Psychodynamics.* London: Butterworths.

Manor, O. (1991) Assessing the work of a family centre. Services offered and referrers' perceptions: A pilot study. *Journal of Family Therapy*, 13, 285–294.

Maslach, C., and Jackson, S. (1982). Burnout in health professions: A social psychological analysis. In G. Sanders and J. Suls (eds) *Social Psychology of Health and Illness.* Hillsdale, NJ: Erlbaum.

Maturana, H. and Varela, F. (1988) *The Tree of Knowledge.* Boston: Shambala.

McCarthy, I. and Byrne, N. (1988) Mistaken love: Conversations on the problem of incest in an Irish context. *Family Process*, 27, 181–199.

McCubbin, H., and Patterson, J. (1991). FILE. In H. McCubbin and A. Thompson (Eds). *Family Assessment Inventories 2nd edition.* Madison, WCN: University of Wisconsin-Madison.

McFarlane, W. (1991) Family psychoeducational treatment. In A. Gurman, and D. Kniskern (eds) *Handbook of Family Therapy. Volume 2.* New York: Brunner/Mazel.

McGoldrick, M. and Gerson, R. (1985) *Genograms in Family Assessment.* New York: Norton.

McGoldrick, M., Anderson, C. and Walsh, F. (1989)*Women in Families: A Framework for family therapy.* New York: Norton.

McGuffin, P. and Gottesman, I. (1985) Genetic influences on normal and abnormal development. In M. Rutter and L. Hersov (eds) *Child and Adolescent Psychiatry. Modern Approaches. 2nd edition.* Oxford: Blackwell.

McKinnon, L. and Miller, D. (1987) The new epistemology and the Milan approach: feminist and socio-political considerations. *Journal of marital and family therapy*, 13, 139–155.

McNamee, S. and Gergen, K. (1991)*Therapy as Social Construction.* London: Sage.

Minuchin, S. (1974) *Families and Family Therapy.* Cambridge, MA: Harvard University Press.

Minuchin, S. and Fishman, H.C. (1981) *Family Therapy Techniques.* Cambridge, MA: Harvard University Press.

Minuchin, S. Rosman, B. and Baker, L. (1978) *Psychosomatic Families: Anorexia Nervosa in Context.* Cambridge, MA: Harvard University Press.

Munton, A. and Stratton, P. (1990) Concepts of causality applied in the clinic: Interactional models and attributional style. *Journal of Cognitive Psychotherapy,* 4, 197–209.

Mussen, P., Conger, J., Kagan, J. and Huston, A. (1990) *Child Development and Personality, 7th edition.* New York: Harper Collins.

Nicol, A., Smith, J., Kay, B., Hall, D., Barlow, J. and Williams, B. (1988) A focused casework approach to the treatment of child abuse: A controlled comparison. *Journal of Child Psychology and Psychiatry,* 29, 703–711.

O'Brien, F. (1939) *At Swim-Two-Birds.* Middlesex: Penguin.

O'Connor, K. (1991)*The play therapy Primer.* New York: Wiley.

Orbach, I. (1988) *Children who don't want to live: Understanding and treating the suicidal child.* San Francisco, CA: Jossy-Bass.

Patterson, G. (1982) *Coercive Family Process.* Eugene, OR: Castalia.

Pimpernell, P., and Treacher, A. (1990) Using a videotape to overcome client's reluctance to engage in family therapy. *Journal of Family Therapy,* 12, 59–71.

Polkinghorne, D. (1992). Post-modern epistemology in practice. In S. Kvale (ed.) *Psychology and Post-modernism.* London: Sage.

Raphael, B. (1984)*The Anatomy of Bereavement.* Hutchinson:London.

Reflection, (1989) Howe's the FT consumer champion. *Context,* 2, 25–26.

Robinson, M. (1991) *Family Transformation Through Divorce and Remarriage.* London: Routledge.

Rutter, M. (1987) Temperament, personality and personality disorder. *British Journal of Psychiatry,* 150, 443–458.

Satir, V. (1967) *Conjoint Family Therapy.* London: Souvenir Press.

Schaeffer, C. and O'Connor, K. (1983) *Handbook of Play Therapy.* New York: Wiley.

Segal, L. (1991) Brief Therapy: The MRI approach. In A. Gurman, and D. Kniskern (eds) *Handbook of Family Therapy. Volume 2.* New York: Brunner/Mazel.

Selvini-Palazzoli, M. (1980) Why a long interval between sessions. In M. Andolfi and I. Zwarling (eds) *Dimensions of Family Therapy.* New York: Guilford.

Selvini-Palazzoli, M. (1985) The problem of the sibling as the referring person. *Journal of Marital and Family Therapy,* 6, 3–9.

Selvini-Palazzoli, M. (1986) Towards a general model of psychotic family games. *Journal of Marital and Family Therapy,* 12, 339–349.

Selvini-Palazzoli, M., Boscolo, L., Cecchin, G. and Prata, G. (1977) Family rituals: A powerful tool in family therapy. *Family Process,* 16, 445–453.

Selvini-Palazzoli, M., Boscolo, L., Cecchin, G. and Prata, G. (1978a) A ritualized prescription in family therapy: Odd days and even days. *Journal of Marital and Family Therapy,* 6, 3–9.

Selvini-Palazzoli, M., Boscolo, L., Cecchin, G. and Prata, G. (1978b) *Paradox and Counterparadox.* New York: Aronson.

Selvini-Palazzoli, M., Boscolo, L., Cecchin, G. and Prata, G. (1980a) Hypothesizing-circularity-neutrality: Three guidelines for the conductor of the session. *Family Process,* 19, 3–12.

Selvini-Palazzoli, M., Boscolo, L., Cecchin, G. and Prata, G. (1980b) The problem of the referring person. *Journal of Marital and Family Therapy,* 11, 31–34.

Selvini-Palazzoli, M., Cirillo, Selvini, M., Sorrentino, A. (1989) *Family Games: General Models of Psychotic Processes within the Family.* New York: Norton.

Selvini-Palazzoli, M. and Prata, G. (1982) Snares in family therapy. *Journal of Marital and Family Therapy,* 8, 443–453.

Shoham-Salomon, V. and Rosenthal, R. (1987) Paradoxical interventions: A meta-analysis. *Journal of Consulting and Clinical Psychology,* 55, 22–27.

Stanton, M and Todd, T. (1982)*The Family Therapy of Drug Abuse and Addiction.* New York: Guilford.

Summit, R. (1983) The child sexual abuse accommodation syndrome. *Child Abuse and Neglect,* 7, 177–193.

Szapocznick, J. et al (1989) Structural family versus-psychodynamic child therapy for problematic Hispanic boys. *Journal of Consulting and Clinical Psychology,* 57, 571–578.

Taylor, S. and Brown, J. (1988) Illusion and well-being: A social psychological perspective on mental health. *Psychological Bulletin,* 103, 193–210.

Thoburn, J. (1988) *Child Placement. Principles and Practice.* Aldershot, Hants: Gower.

Tomm, K. (1984a) One Perspective on the Milan Systemic Approach. Part 1. Overview of Development, Theory and Practice. *Journal of Marital and Family Therapy,* 10, 113–125.

Tomm, K. (1984b) One Perspective on the Milan Systemic Approach. Part 11. Description of session format, interviewing style and interventions. *Journal of Marital and Family Therapy,* 10, 253–271.

Tomm, K. (1987a) Interventive Interviewing Part 1. Strategising as a fourth guideline for the therapist. *Family Process,* 25, 4–13.

Tomm, K. (1987b) Interventive Interviewing Part 11. Reflexive questioning as a means to enable self healing. *Family Process,* 26, 167–183.

Tomm, K. (1988) Interventive Interviewing Part 111. Intending to ask linear, circular, strategic or reflexive questions. *Family Process,* 27, 1–15.

Tomm, K. (1991) *Ethical postures in therapy. Facilitating clients empowerment.* Workshop held at Lambeth Teachers Centre, Lawn Lane, Vauxhall, London under the auspices of Kensington Consultation Centre, 19th and 20th November, 1991.

Tomm, K. and Wright, L. (1979) Training in family therapy: Perceptual, conceptual and executive skills. *Family Process,* 18, 227–250.

Ursano, R. and Hales, R. (1986) A review of brief individual psychotherapies. *American Journal of Psychiatry,* 143, 1507–1517.

Walker, A. (1985) Reconceptualizing family stress. *Journal of Marriage and the Family,* November, 827–837.

Walsh, F. (1993) *Normal Family Processes. 2nd edition.* New York: Guilford.

Watzlawick, P. Weakland, J. and Fisch, R. (1974) *Change.* New York. Norton.

Weeks, G. and L'Abate, L. (1982) *Paradoxical Psychotherapy.* New York: Brunner/Mazel.

Wehr, T. and Rosenthal, N. (1989) Seasonality and affective illness. *American Journal of Psychiatry,* 146, 829–839.

Wendorf, D. and Wendorf, R. (1985) A systemic view of family therapy ethics. *Family Process,* 24, 443–460.

White, M. (1993) Deconstruction and therapy. In S. Gilligan and R. Price (eds.) *Therapeutic Conversations.* New York: Norton.

White, M. and Epston, D. (1990) *Narrative Means to Therapeutic Ends.* New York: Norton.

Willbach, D. (1989) Ethics and family therapy: The case management of family violence. *Journal of Marital and Family Therapy,* 15, 43–52.

Wolkind, S. and Rutter, M. (1985) Separation, loss and Family Relationships. In M. Rutter and L. Hersov (eds.). *Child and Adolescent Psychiatry. Modern Approaches. 2nd. edition.* Oxford: Blackwell.

Woody, J. (1990) Resolving ethical concerns in clinical practice: Toward a pragmatic model. *Journal of Marital and Family Therapy,* 16, 133–150.

World Health Organization (1992) *The ICD-10 Classification of Mental and Behavioural Disorders.* Geneva: WHO.

Wynne, L. McDaniel, S. and Weber, T. (1986) *Systems Consultation: A New Perspective for Family Therapy.* New York: Guilford.

Zygmond, M. and Boorhem, H. (1989) Ethical decision making in family therapy. *Family Process,* 28, 269–280.

Index